D0923340

CATARACT
GLAUCOMA
AND OTHER EYE DISORDERS

CATARACT

GLAUCOMA

AND OTHER EYE DISORDERS

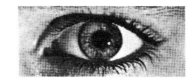

PREVENTION

AND

CURE

WITH PROVEN NATURAL METHODS

BY
JOHN H.
TOBE

First Printing August, 1973
Second Printing September, 1973

Printed in Canada

TABLE OF CONTENTS

ILLUSTRATIONS

Introduction

Why would a layman attempt to write a book on cataract? That question was actually asked of me when I mentioned to various individuals that I was doing a book on the subject. My reply was direct . . . "Simply because honest information on cataract is sorely lacking and badly needed."

Meaningful literature on any health topic was scarce or nonexistent until the last few decades. Granted, there are many books and papers dealing with cataracts, glaucoma and various eye disorders but they are of little value to the layman or as we say 'John Smith'. Yes, there are scads of pamphlets and even books sponsored and published by the drug or optical lens manufacturers but they have a motive and that motive is not in the best interests of John Smith. Sales motivation when involved with health should be a prime No-No, but in our dollar oriented society what can we do?

The dairy industry, the meat industry, the gelatin manufacturers, the optical companies, the chemical companies, etc., etc. have access to promotion via Madison Avenue, the printing press, authors and publishers, newspapers, magazines, radio and television, so thus honest writing, reporting, researching and publishing are hard to find. That is my main, foremost reason for writing this book. It is not even necessary that I make money — because I have a private income — I need only cover expenses. My motive is to reveal the causes of poor or failing vision and blindness in young and old. Whether you believe me or not is your problem . . . you will have to decide for yourself.

Besides this, I am concerned about my health, my eyes and all my organs and in my selfishness I set myself a spartan way of life so that I can remain in good health — but I am unselfish enough to pass this life-saving information on to those who trust me.

For more than 15 years I have been gathering information on cataract. I believe I have covered every known source of information. I am still sifting cogent data as the book goes to press. Apart from my reading, inquiring and searching I wrote hundreds of letters to experts and practitioners in all the healing fields in all parts of the world. I also wrote to individuals, sufferers, those who have had cataract surgery as well as those who have tried other methods . . . anyone whom I felt, or had heard, had some knowledge about cataract.

When I started to inquire and gather information on cataracts and glaucoma I was more than surprised to learn that information on cataracts and glaucoma was not only scanty but downright fragmentary. With a condition as serious and important as cataract or glaucoma one would think that details concerning cause, effect, methods of treatment and cure, if any, would be voluminous. Instead, the actual medical information pertaining to cause, effect, etc., would barely make a good sized pamphlet. Besides, it is mainly repetitious, everybody repeating everybody else.

However, my method of unearthing or extracting information does not restrict itself to the normal channels. I use virtually "any" source . . . scientific, empirical, as well as folk lore, old wives' tales, personal experiences, even the 'I have a friend, who has a friend who told, etc.'

Some of the best and most reliable information came from actual sufferers, patients who had undergone the ordeal from A to Z, who told their story honestly and without coaching, prodding or prompting.

Admittedly, I have run into problems with this book, problems due to the fact that there seems to be a curtain surrounding cataract information. Nobody seems to know anything about cataract. From the medical records I can get volumes and volumes of data and such but as far as discovering anything concerning the cause or the cure without surgery they give absolutely nothing. The medical fraternity and the optical associations and corporations claim most vociferously and repeatedly over and over and over again that there is no known cause of senile cataract. It would appear that they are trying to convince themselves.

I contend that it doesn't make sense for a condition to exist without cause. My studies have revealed that no condition and no event occurs on this earth without cause. Why do some people who reach 90 and 100 go through their lives with hardly any impairment of their vision while others begin to have trouble and show signs of cataract development in their 30's, 40's and 50's? Also, why do we find congenital and other forms of cataract in infancy and childhood?

The medical profession treats cataract lightly, as though it were of no great consequence. They just say "Oh, wait until the cataracts are fully ripened or developed and then we'll remove them and that will be the end of your problem".

I suggest that is the most misleading statement ever made, if not a deliberate, downright lie . . . a brutal, devastating lie. I claim that surgery is just the beginning of the problem because they don't actually tell you that you are comparatively blind without the special glasses with which they supply you for a fixed sum and even then your vision is not very good. I learned this from actual conversation with virtually hundreds of people who have had cataract surgery. If I have learned nothing else from my studies I'm definitely convinced that surgery is not the answer for cataract and that it should be avoided if humanly possible. A similar situation exists with glaucoma.

The important thing about this work on cataract is that I have definitely found various ways and means by which (a) cataract can be prevented, (b) cataract can be slowed, (c) cataract advance can be stopped, (d) cataract can be made to recede, (e) cataract can be cured where opacity is not complete.

When I first set out to do the book and was gathering information I faced the simple truth that I probably would not find a way or means of curing or coping with the condition. However, as the evidence began to come in and accumulate I saw then that cataract need not be the fearful monster that it is — that there were logical, sane ways of making the condition disappear and also a comparatively simple means of preventing it from happening.

Therefore, in reading this book you will find that not only can you stop the growth of cataracts immediately but in a few short months you can make them recede or disappear, unless the condition has been permitted to advance to an irreversible condition. Like everyone else in

America I previously believed that the only answer to cataract was to go to an optometrist, physician or ophthalmologist who would send you to a surgeon and have the cataract removed when it was ready. I accepted this up until a few years ago . . . in fact, up until I began to gather evidence . . . then I found out that cataracts need not be feared because they can be controlled and they can be corrected without drugs, surgery or irradiation.

I cite this data as my qualification to write this book.

1 Physiology of the Eye

PARTS OF THE EYE

I felt that it would be advisable to give some information on the eye and explain the various terms that are generally used. I realize that most people know what a lens or a retina is but still in order to avoid any misunderstanding and also to make it clear to you without any searching on your part I thought I'd better cover the situation here.

The eyeball is a sphere, approximately 1 inch in diameter with a pronounced bulge on its outer surface, the walls of which consist of three distinct layers or coats and the contents of which are about 95 percent liquid. Of these three coats, the outer one gives the eye its shape and furnishes protection, the intermediate coat serves chiefly to provide nutrition, and the inmost coat, or layer, contains the all-important sight cells.

The **sclera** is the outer layer which also acts as a protective coating for the eyeball and it is usually known as

1

the 'white' of the eye. The middle layer coating of the eye is known as the **choroid** which is a vascular layer lining the posterior 3/5th of the eyeball. The choroid is continuous with the **ciliary body** and with the **iris** which lies at the front of the eye. Now we come to the innermost layer which is light-sensitive and is called the **retina.**

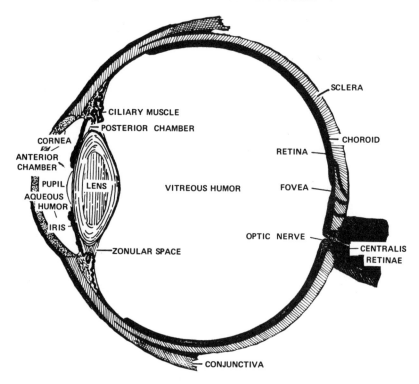

The **cornea** is a tough, five-layered membrane and it is through this membrane that light is admitted to the interior of the eye. The **aqueous humor** is found behind the cornea and is a chamber filled with clear, watery fluid and this separates the cornea from the **crystalline lens.** The crystalline lens is a flattened sphere constructed of a large number of transparent fibers arranged in layers, which is connected by ligaments to a ringlike muscle, called the **ciliary muscle,** which surrounds it. It is due to the ciliary body or muscle that the lens is flattened or curved as is

2

required to change the focal length and this enables the eye to focus sharply on distant or nearby objects. This is referred to as accommodation and in this there is some controversy as mentioned elsewhere in this book.

Behind the cornea and in front of the lens we find the **pigmented iris.** It has a circular opening in its center. It is this opening which we know as the **pupil** and it is controlled by a muscle around its edge. It is this muscle which contracts or relaxes, making the pupil larger or smaller, to control the amount of light admitted to the eye.

The **vitreous humor** is a transparent, jellylike substance which is found behind the lens and which fills the main body of the eye. It is the pressure of the vitreous humor and the aqueous humor which keeps the eyeball distended.

The **retina** is a complex layer, composed largely of nerve cells. The light-sensitive receptor cells lie on the outer surface of the retina in front of a **pigmented tissue layer.**

The **rods and cones** are types of light sensitive cells so named because they resemble rods and cones when viewed through a powerful microscope. The rods react to dim light and the movement of objects. The cones are the cells that enable us to see color and fine detail.

The **macula lutea** is found directly behind the pupil and it is a small yellow pigmented spot in the center of which is the **fovea centralis.** The fovea centralis is the area of greatest visual acuity of the eye. The **sensory layer** is found at the center of the fovea and is composed entirely of cone-shaped cells.

The **optic nerve** is found at the entrance to the eyeball. Below and slightly to the inner side of the fovea there is a small round area of the retina which has no light-sensitive cells. This is known as the **optic disc** and forms the blind spot of the eye.

Now let us discuss some of the protective structures.

The **eyelids** are composed of two folds of skin and tissue, upper and lower, which can be closed by means of muscles to form a protective covering over the eyeball. This affords protection against excessive light and mechanical injury.

The **eyelashes,** which are composed of a fringe of short hairs growing on the edge of either eyelid, act as a screen to keep dust particles and insects out of the eyes when the eyelids are partly closed. The **conjunctiva** is found inside the eyelids and is composed of a thin protective membrane, which doubles over to cover the visible sclera. Each eye is equipped with a **tear gland** or as it is properly known, a **lachrimal organ** which is situated at the outside corner of the eye. These glands excrete a salty secretion which lubricates the forward part of the eyeball when the eyelids are closed and flushes away any small dust particles or various other foreign matter which may appear on the surface of the eye.

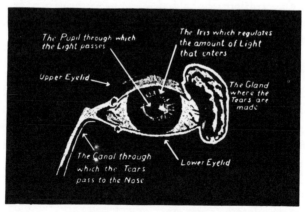

Frontal View Of The Eye

The **meibomian glands** are found on the edges of the eyelids and are a number of small glands which produce a fatty secretion that lubricates the eyelids themselves and the eyelashes.

The **eyebrows** are located above each eye and appear to have a protective function which consists mainly of soaking up or deflecting perspiration or rain and preventing the moisture from running into the eyes.

The **socket** is the aperature in the skull in which the eye is set. It is referred to as the **orbit**. The bony edges of the orbit, as well as the frontal bone, and the cheekbone protect the eye from mechanical injury by physical blows or accidents and collisions.

HOW THE EYE WORKS

The following is a very good description by a leading optical company on exactly how the eye works for us.

"Because light bends, it can carry information to the eye. For instance, we see a man ten feet in front of us because the light surrounding him is bounced and bent out of the way (reflected) by his body. If it could pass through him he would be invisible.

"Seeing begins with light entering the eye and bringing with it the information it has picked up in touching the objects in its path. The light patterns travel through the various parts of the eye until the image is cast upon the back wall, or retina, of the eye just as a picture is transferred to film by a camera.

"But getting a clear, intact image to the retina is no simple matter. First, the amount of light entering the eye must be regulated. Then the image must be focused sharply on the retina, as a subject must be focused on film to make a good picture.

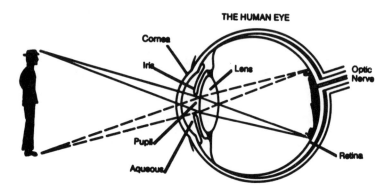

THE HUMAN EYE

How The Eye Works

"Controlling the amount of light that enters the eye is done solely by the iris, which has the eye's coloring — blue, brown, gray or green. This iris is a diaphragm made up largely of circular and radiating muscles. These muscles, by contracting and stretching, are able to shrink or enlarge the size of the light admitting hole, the pupil.

"The tasks of controlling and focusing light are performed by a delicately engineered system which includes the parts shown and labeled in the diagram. The **cornea,** a transparent tissue rising from the opaque white of the eye, bends light. Behind the cornea is a clear fluid called the **aqueous humor,** which also plays a part in focusing. Next in order is the donut-shaped **iris,** with its hole, the **pupil,** lying almost directly in line with the cornea.

"After the light has passed through the cornea, aqueous humor and pupil, it goes through the **lens.** The **ciliary muscles** alter the shape of the lens, making it more or less convex to provide focusing for near and far viewing. The light proceeds through a jellylike substance known as

6

the **vitreous humor** and reaches the **retina,** the light-sensitive lining around the inside of the eye.

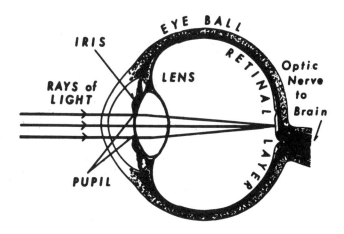

The Normal Eye

"In the retina are the two types of light-sensitive cells called 'rods' and 'cones'. The rods react to dim light and movement of objects. The cones enable one to see color and fine detail, and are especially concentrated in and near the **fovea,** a slight depression in the retina at the back of the eye.

"When light falls on the rod and cone cells, a chemical change takes place which touches off impulses that travel through the **optic nerve** to the brain. Here the patterns of impulses combine to produce the visual experience of an image."

WHAT IS 20/20 VISION?

Here we have the views of an optical company concerning the definition of 20/20 vision.

"It is a way of stating that visual acuity (acuteness or sharpness of vision) is normal. Literally, it means that at 20

7

feet a person sees the size of letters on the examination chart that he is supposed to see at 20 feet. If, at this 20-foot distance, a person can only read letters of the size normally read at a distance of 40 feet, he is said to have 20/40 visual acuity (V.A.). Thus, the larger the bottom number of the fraction, the more blurred the vision. Some people have better than normal acuity and this is indicated by a smaller bottom number, such as 20/15."

2 What is Cataract?

Cataract is the most common cause of blindness in America today. Cataract occurs when the crystalline lens of the eye becomes increasingly clouded or opaque. Vision is gradually diminished as the opacity increases. This condition progresses if no action is taken until the point of blindness. Usually when this happens surgical treatment is advised by most medical physicians and surgeons. The medical profession knows no other means of treatment nor does it recommend any other means of treatment. The medical-surgery treatment is the removal of the crystalline lens. This, according to medical propaganda, restores good vision an estimated 95 percent of the time. This is not borne out by investigation.

The simplest description of cataract is "the opacity of lens of the eye or its capsule or both, which may be developmental or degenerative." Now the difference between developmental cataract and degenerative cataract is that developmental cataract occurs congenitally or during early life as a result of heredity and nutritional or inflammatory disturbances whereas degenerative cataract is characterized by gradual loss of transparency in a normally developed lens. This may be due to senile degenerative changes, the effects of heat, X ray irradiation, trauma, systemic disorders — for example, diabetes, uveal tract inflammation (which is complicated cataract) and ingestion of certain toxic substances, for example drugs.

The word cataract is used to describe the condition of the opacification of the crystalline lens of the eye. The origin of the word cataract stems from the erroneous belief that a cataract consisted of a kind of curtain which fell down like a waterfall inside the eye, obscuring the pupil. Then it was believed that the humour of the brain was falling down over the pupil.

It appears that cataract affects mostly middle-aged and older people. However, let it not be thought that cataract does not strike the young because it does and it can affect a person at any age. However, the congenital variety is the most common cause of cataract in young people.

An eminent authority on cataract and the eyes described cataract as follows:

"Simply dormant or dead cells found in the crystalline lens of the eye. The grayer-whiter they are, the more advanced the condition." He further describes the crystalline lens as 'a body of cells hanging suspended by ligaments just behind the iris of the eye, has a layered structure similar to that seen when an onion is cut in half.'

"The cells composing its layered mass, unlike those found elsewhere in the body where a capillary is never more than one additional cell away, have no capillaries at all. These cells get their daily bread and their metabolic wastes discharged by a specialized process which reminds me of the flow of wax of a candle wick in the direction of the flame. This must be because the presence of blood vessels in the structure would block the passage of light through it. The lens is clear in health, resembling the clear part of one's fingernails.

"Such a circulation method is highly specialized and with specialization comes hazard, since the lens cells become highly vulnerable to any nutritional interference or to their waste removal. They are a weak link in the body chain."

According to investigators there are over 150 kinds of cataract or lens opacities but we will just mention the leading 6 systematically grouped divisions.

Developmental Cataract — In which some defect during growth, either hereditary, nutritional, or inflammatory, has affected the normal growth of lens fibres, with consequent loss of transparency. In this group are included the congenital forms of posterior polar cataract, anterior polar cataract, central cataract, lamellar or zonular cataract, coronary and punctate cataract, and complete congenital and juvenile cataract.

Degenerative Cataract — In which normally developed lens substance loses its transparency as the result of degenerative changes. This group comprises the commonest variety of cataract — i.e. senile nuclear and cortical cataract.

Traumatic Cataract — Due to a perforating injury or severe contusion.

Irradiation Cataract — Due to exposure to certain rays.

Complicated Cataract — Due to some other ocular disease.

Cataract associated with Systemic Disease and Poisons.

Cataract can also be grouped or sub-grouped, according to the part of the lens involved, into (1) capsular, (2) capsulolenticular, or (3) lenticular cataract; or according as they are (1) progressive (degenerative cataract is usually progressive) or (2) stationary (developmental cataract is usually stationary).

PATHOLOGY OF CATARACT

The earliest change in a lens which is becoming opaque is the accumulation of fluid between the fibers forming rounded bodies called Morgagnian globules. When this occurs the lens fibers swell and break down to form irregular masses of debris. These changes affect the cortex. In some cases the whole cortex is liquified, leaving the nucleus unchanged. This is referred to or known as a Morgagnian cataract.

The function of the lens is to focus the luminous rays so that they form a perfect image on the retina. To accomplish this the refractive power of the lens must change with the distance of the object, according to whether the light rays are parallel or divergent. This alteration in the refractive power of the lens is known as accommodation and is produced by a change of shape affecting mainly its anterior curvature. In old age the lens increases in size, is flattened and assumes a yellow tinge becoming tougher and less transparent. This process of sclerosis accounts for the gray reflection seen in the pupil of the aged, which may be mistaken for cataract. It also explains the inability of the part of the lens of a person of advanced years to change its shape for the purpose of accommodation.

Congenital cataract may arise from delayed formation of the anterior chamber and contact of the lens with the cornea during foetal life and it is as a rule bilateral. On occasions there may be an opacity in the anterior cortex separated from the capsular opacity by a clear lens substance which has developed after the original opacity was formed (reduplication cataract).

By far the most frequent variety of cataract in children is lamellar or zonular cataract. It almost invariably affects both eyes. It is due to some hereditary malfunction or nutritional deficiency during the process of development, which causes the layer of the lens substance formed during that period to develop abnormally. It is said to be accompanied sometimes by signs of rickets; the enamel of the permanent teeth may be affected by the same nutritional disturbance. The cataract consists of a gray, disc-like opacity of the layer surrounding the transparent nucleus with clear cortex on the outside.

By far the most prevalent type of cataract in adults is referred to as degenerative cataract or senile cataract. It is generally claimed to be an affliction of advanced life. However, it is sometimes seen as early as 40 years of age and there definitely appears to be a familial tendency to cataract in which case the condition may occur at even an earlier age in subsequent generations.

As a rule both eyes are involved but frequently one in advance of the other. The opacity may begin either in a superficial part of the cortex or in the part immediately surrounding the nucleus. Senile cataract involves the cortex, the nucleus remaining transparent throughout the process. The time required for full development varies greatly. It may ripen completely in a few months, or may require many years to develop. It may become stationary at any stage of its progress.

Now let us discuss the function of the crystalline lens which is the part of the eye that goes hay-wire and is the part of the organ that is affected or causes cataract. It is a completely bloodless organ or part of an organ having no direct contact with the circulatory system of the body. This is an important consideration. The crystalline lens of the eye is not fed directly by your blood stream or by nerves, arteries or capillaries. It is surrounded within the eye by the aqueous humour produced by the ciliary bodies which is a water-like fluid that fills the anterior third of the eyeball. The aqueous humour is directly linked with the blood stream and it supplies nutrients to the lens. It is interference with the supply of nutrients that causes the lens to become cloudy and lose its transparency.

Frequently a serious involvement occurs when the cataract in one eye has become troublesome enough to interfere with vision while the other eye is comparatively functional. Under such circumstances only one eye is operated upon. Then the proper glasses containing the mechanical lens cannot be fitted as you can clearly understand and this leads to considerable indecision. Personally, I would hate to be put in that predicament . . . that is, to have to decide whether or not to operate upon or involve an eye that is still generally functionable. So it's a toss up as to whether or not you wait until the other eye becomes clouded with cataract so that both eyes can be operated on at the same time.

However, not all individuals are involved to the same degree. For example, a man in a home for the aged or one who does just a bit of gardening or ordinary household or home duties is not in the same position as a man who studies or reads or is in a business, profession or trade that requires continued use of the eyes in a more or less concentrated way. The former can wait until both eyes are affected and then have them both operated on and the glasses and lens fitted accordingly. However, the individual who depends upon his eyesight for practically everything, including his livelihood, has a very difficult decision to

14

make because here he can still see and get by with one eye but he has to sacrifice the good eye in order to have the surgery done and the glasses fitted. So you can see this creates a traumatic situation. The individual in the first category may never need to worry about it because the situation may never get to the stage where he is comparatively visionless.

I personally have known many people in my lifetime who had cataracts and yet in their general farm work or gardening work it was not serious enough for them to even desire to have an operation. Sure, their vision was cloudy and foggy and they sometimes stumbled about a bit but they were of advanced age and felt that this was better than becoming irreversibly blind which was the fear they had if they were operated on and the operation wasn't successful. So you see it depends a great deal upon how much you use or how much you depend upon your eyes.

Surgeons claim that the removal of the senile cataract is a simple procedure that is, in their opinion, absolutely safe. From the literature that I have read and from the stories that have been told to me by people who have had surgery the picture is by no means so well defined. In some cases it was rather easy with a very quick recovery whereas with others it was a prolonged, serious, troublesome, drawn-out affair with a great deal of trauma being involved. Of course this could be affected by the individual's make-up and character as well as the work and skill of the surgeon. As one expert described it . . . the operation is frequently done under local anesthesia and the patient is frequently out of bed in a very few days.

In cataract surgery the lens must be removed from inside the eye and then a substitute lens must be supplied in the glasses that you wear forever after if you are to have any worthwhile vision at all.

Dr. David O. Harrington, writing in the American Journal of Ophthalmology, claims that "Many disturbances and diseases of the eye are wholly or partly psychogenic (this means caused by the mind). He suggests that greater attention should be paid to emotional problems when seeking a cure."

Glaucoma is said to be due to defective circulation in the vessels that supply blood and nutrients to the eyes. Because circulation is controlled by the central nervous system, emotional conflict and problems may affect the eyes. To have good eye health you must have good body health.

The onset of cataract as well as other visual problems is claimed to be complicated by cholesterol narrowing the passageways of the blood ... the arteries. When in experiments cholesterol levels have been brought down vision has been known to have improved. Vitamin D is involved in calcium assimilation and proper calcium assimilation is essential if one is to have good vision. I suggest that natural vitamin D from food sources, or better still from sunlight and the atmosphere, is essential or important for calcium metabolization and this will help prevent cataracts.

Eye conditions are probably the most serious that can face a human being. Cancer, heart disease, arthritis and many other diseases are bad, very bad but when it comes to the threat of losing one's eyesight I doubt if much can be worse. I know many people would choose death rather than be blind. In fact, I've come across in my studies many stories of people who, after their cataract surgery upon finding that they couldn't see nearly as well as was promised, hardly at all or were practically blind or were doomed to blindness, committed suicide. There are more of these cases than are generally recognized.

All the healing professions recommend drugs, palliations, treatments, eyeglasses, surgery and contact lenses but practically nobody suggests a healthy body and proper nutrition. I want to stress here now, clearly and unmistakably, that 95 percent of eye troubles in America are based on nutrition, stress, or emotions. As shocking as it may sound to you I repeat, that 95 percent of all the eye troubles in America are caused by poor diet and stress. Therefore, if these are the causes then removing these causes or correcting them should cause the condition to disappear. Yes, that is precisely what I'm saying.

The next statement from you may be "Then you suggest that all the ophthalmologists and all the physicians and all the surgeons and all the other various healers in the world are wrong, are mistaken and you are right."

My reply is, "I call the score as I see it and that is what I see." You will find by my bibliography that I have examined, studied, investigated and researched to a fairly great degree, apart from my personal discussions and investigations. I want to make my position unmistakably clear for the record so that there will be no confusion regarding my stand and viewpoint. If any drug or drugs, herb, surgery or any concoction on the face of the earth were found to help one restore or maintain vision I would be all for it. I don't care how unconventional, how orthodox or how unorthodox it might be, I would support it with all my strength and my pen as soon as it were proven or established. While I am a naturist and believe strongly or completely in nature, if you can show me that the devil or any power or any healer on earth has the means and method of helping people see better or correcting their visional faults, I'll support it. All I need is the proof. In my quest for truth I shake my prejudices and state that I am not anti-medicine nor anti-surgery, nor anti-chiropractic nor anti-osteopathic, anti-homeopathic or against any other form of healing. I just want the best for you.

You cannot have a sick mind and a healthy body. They must both be healthy. You cannot have sick eyes in a healthy body. It is impossible, unless by injury. Even then the body is no longer well if the eyes are sick.

Now this principle is not new. At this stage let me quote "Intransparency of the crystalline lens is technically known as cataract. Cataract may be idiopathic and uncomplicated or traumatic or secondary to disease in the deeper part of the eye. The modified epithelial structure of which the lens is composed is always being added to throughout life. The older portions of the lens are consequently the more central. They are harder and less elastic. This arrangement seems to predispose the difficulties of nutrition. In many people, in the absence altogether of general or local disease, the transparency of the lens is lost owing to degeneration of the incompletely nourished fibers. This idiopathic cataract mostly occurs in old people; hence the term senile cataract. So-called senile cataract is not, however, necessarily associated with any general senile change."

I have a very definite purpose in quoting the above. It is from the Encyclopedia Britannica, page 97, Vol. 10, 11th Edition. It was published in 1910 and was probably seven or more years in preparation. This means that nutrition has been recognized as a factor in cataract for approximately 70 years.

In another place let me quote "Often it is advisable to do something for general health". Another quote, "It is a common and dangerous mistake to overtreat."

Therefore, it is clear that 70 or more years ago the medical profession knew that nutrition was a factor in cataract and specifically, that the structure of the lens must be nourished and fed or as I express it, it must be continually cellularly regenerated. Today it is seldom even suggested or mentioned that nutrition could be a factor in cataract, glaucoma or other afflictions or diseases of the eye.

It is high time that the medical profession, ophthalmologists, optometrists and opticians stopped shoring up the Helmholtz theory. More than 115 years ago Herman Ludwig Ferdinand Von Helmholtz, a great philosopher, man of science, medical doctor, the man who invented the ophthalmometer or ophthalmoscope, came up with the theory of accommodation on which orthodox ophthalmology is still based. He claimed that accommodation is effected by the change in shape of the lens. In turn this change is governed by the action of the ciliary muscles, although he did not offer any reasonable explanation as to how the ciliary muscles operated and he also admitted that his theory was merely a probability because the image obtained on the lens was so variable and uncertain that to use his own words it is "most usually so blurred that the form of the flame could not be definitely distinguished."

It was Helmholtz who came up with the theory that nearsightedness and farsightedness, as well as most other errors of refraction, were fixed states, that these conditions could not be corrected. He believed that somewhere along the line either through birth or other reason these faults existed and there was no cure for the situation and the only means of help was to wear artificial lenses so ground as to counteract the refractive error of the crystalline lens. From that day to the present day the entire medical profession and the various branches that deal with the eyes and vision, such as ophthalmologists, opticians and optometrists have accepted and followed that principle. Millions upon millions of people in America today wear glasses because of Helmholtz's illogical theory and millions have become blind because of this theory and the whole field of vision still clings to it and refuses to see the light and make changes.

It was Dr. William Horatio Bates, an ophthalmologist himself, who annually examined more than 30,000 pairs of eyes at the Eye And Ear Infirmary in New York, who began to question the validity of Helmholtz's theory. Poor Dr. Bates, in spite of all the marvelous work he did, was ridiculed, harassed and persecuted but he did not work in vain . . . hundreds of thousands have benefitted from his legacy.

I'm suggesting to my readers that they investigate for themselves and weigh the validity of the Helmholtz theory against the statements of Dr. Bates and other qualified writers who maintain that errors of refraction can be corrected without the use of crippling glasses.

3 Signs and Symptoms of Cataract

There are several recognized signs or symptoms of cataract. Some persons having one or even all of them may not necessarily have cataract, but their presence indicates the need for a thorough visual examination by an eye physician.

1. Blurred vision is one of the first signs of trouble. The cataract patient finds it impossible to see things as clearly as he once did. Since less light can now reach the retina, the person may find he must hold objects closer to his eye than before. He may complain of being unable to find a light bright enough to read by. Sometimes diplopia (double vision) occurs due to irregular refraction of the lens. The irregular refraction may also cause discomfort due to glare. Myopia (near-sightedness) often develops during the early stages, due to increased density and refractive power of the lens. (This is referred to as lenticular myopia). For this reason the patient may be able to discard his reading glasses for the time, but he may need concave spherical glasses for distant vision.

2. Double vision or spots may occupy a fixed position in the visual field as the cataract progresses. Lights in particular may appear double; a person looking at the moon or a street light may not see it clearly outlined but as if there were two or more.

3. Changing eyeglasses frequently indicates the possibility of a cataract near the center of the lens.

4. There is a diminished acuteness of vision, depending upon the situation and the kind of cataract. It is greatest when the opacity is central and diffuse, and least when the cataract is peripheral. When central, the patient sees best in dim light — with dilatation of the pupil. The interference with vision increases with the progress of the cataract, until finally there is mere perception of light.

5. The pupil of the eye, which normally appears black, takes on a milky gray or whitish color. Usually the

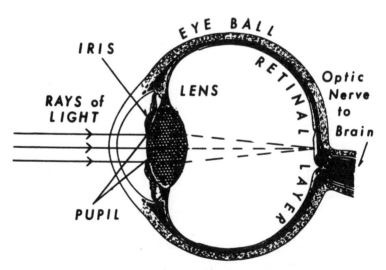

Rays of light blocked; only a few scattered rays pass through Cataract Lens.

cataract patient is not able to detect this change in the pupil by himself. This one sign is more readily detected by the doctor or companions of the patient than by the cataract victim himself.

There are no inflammatory symptoms. Examination by oblique illumination shows a grayish or whitish opacity on a black ground, and with the ophthalmoscope at a distance a black opacity upon a red background. The pupil should be dilated with a mydriatic in order that the lens and the fundus may be examined. During the stage of swelling of a complete cataract the anterior chamber is reduced in depth. This swelling of the lens may cause increase of tension in an eye predisposed to glaucoma.

There are four stages of cataract: Incipient Stage, Maturing Stage, Mature Stage, Hypermature Stage.

Incipient Stage: The opacity most frequently begins as streaks, starting from the periphery of the cortex where they are wider, and then extending to the centre of the lens, where they narrow like the spokes of a wheel. These streaks appear grayish by oblique illumination, and black when seen with the ophthalmoscope. Between these sectors the lens is transparent. Less frequently, senile cataract begins with dot-like or cloud-like opacities situated in any portion of the lens. Sometimes the portion immediately surrounding the nucleus becomes opaque, constituting so-called nuclear cataract. The last form causes a relatively large amount of visual disturbance. Cataract sometimes remains stationary in the incipient stage for an indefinite period, with little impairment of vision.

The stage of Swelling (maturing or developing stage): The lens absorbs an increasing amount of fluid, swells, and by pushing the iris forward reduces the depth of the anterior chamber. It appears bluish-white, shining, and presents distinctly the markings of the stellate figure.

23

During this stage the iris casts a shadow upon the lens when the eye is illuminated from the side, since the superficial portion of the lens is still transparent, the opaque layer being some distance behind the iris.

Mature Stage: The lens loses most of its fluid, shrinks somewhat, and becomes opaque and of a dull gray or amber colour, the stellate markings still being recognizable. The anterior chamber regains its normal depth, and there is no shadow thrown by the iris on the lens with focal illumination. Occasionally the entire lens is changed into a hard, dark brown mass (black cataract). In this stage the cataract can easily be separated from the capsule of the lens. It is then said to be 'ripe' for operation, since it can be extracted whole by the extra-capsular method without leaving any portion of the cortex behind.

Hypermature Stage: The cataract may continue in the mature stage for a considerable time. If changes continue, the surface of the lens loses its radial markings and becomes homogeneous, or presents irregular spots. The lens may continue to lose water, and thus a shrunken, flattened mass results (shrunken cataract), with some deepening of the anterior chamber. Or, the cortex may become soft, liquid, and milky, and the nucleus sink to the bottom of the capsule (Morgagnian cataract), the cataract appearing white with a brownish colouring below. Old hypermature cataracts often contain deposits of cholesterol or of lime-salts. The latter change (chalky cataract) is found chiefly in complicated cataracts. The anterior capsule may become thickened and opaque (capsulolenticular cataract). The lens (and iris) may become tremulous through stretching of the suspensory ligament. For these reasons operation on a cataract in the over-ripe stage is often less favourable and more difficult than during the mature period.

The foremost symptom is a gradual diminution of

visual acuity. The degree of visional loss is dependent upon the location and the extent of the opacity. Well developed diffuse cataract may reduce vision until only light perception and projection remain. In the early stages of nuclear cataracts myopia often develops. In this manner an older person may discover that he can read without his glasses and this is referred to as second sight.

It is a fact that when cataract is well advanced it can be seen with the unaided eye as a gray opacity in the lens. However, under examination by an ophthalmologist the cataract can be seen in its earlier stages of development. A small cataract can be seen under close examination as dark defects in the red reflex. Gradual loss of vision in middle-aged or older patients is characteristic of both cataract and glaucoma. Medical authorities and the consensus of medical opinion and medical texts and literature tell us that the vision lost through cataract is restored by operation, but the deterioration due to glaucoma, mistakenly diagnosed as cataract, may result in permanent blindness. Therefore, glaucoma must first be ruled out in every case.

CHEMICAL CHANGES THAT TAKE PLACE IN EXPERIMENTAL CATARACT

"Increase In Water — There is a relative increase in water, which disappears gradually as the cataract becomes mature. The total amount of water eventually decreases, and at the same time the weight of the lens diminishes.

"Increase In The Percentage Of Ash — The nucleus is said to contain a greater percentage of ash than the cortex after cataract formation. (1, 2)

"Increase In Sodium — It has already been stated that the potassium-sodium ratio may be taken as an index of tissue vitality. (1, 3) In the normal cortex this ratio equals

1.65 and in the nucleus, 1.34. In cataract this falls to 0.41 in the cortex and 0.32 in the nucleus because of the rise in sodium and the fall in potassium.

"Decrease In Potassium — Potassium decreases sharply, dropping from 21.8 percent in the ash of normal lenses to 8.45 percent in mature cataract. *(4)* There is a loss of potassium in almost all forms of experimental cataract. In galactose cataract, the potassium falls from 0.222 percent wet weight in normal lenses to 0.165 percent in the cataractous lens. *(5)* The loss of potassium is probably caused by the breakdown of complexes of organic potassium, after which the potassium diffuses away from the lens. This probably indicates death of the cell. At the same time, the loss of potassium permits sodium to penetrate into the lens fibers and accounts for the increased sodium content of cataractous lenses. The potassium content decreases in traumatic cataract and in cataract following experimental parathyroidectomy.

"Increase In Calcium Content — The calcium content increases. This is not a primary change in the cataractous process, however, since Bellows has shown that, in galactose cataract, the calcium deposition follows the primary cataractous changes. The increased calcium content has always been of interest because cataract develops in man and in experimental animals when the normal calcium relationships of the body are disturbed in conditions such as rickets and following parathyroidectomy. In normal lenses the ash contains 1 percent calcium, in immature cataract it contains 2.3 percent, and in mature cataract it contains 5.5 percent. This relationship between calcium content and stage of maturity is so intimate that Salit classifies cataracts on this basis. Those whose calcium content is below 10 mg./100 gm. (wet weight) are classified as incipient, those with a calcium content from 10 to 35 mg./100 gm. as immature, and those with a calcium content above 35 mg./100 gm. as mature.

"Decrease In Oxygen Consumption — The oxygen consumption of the lens decreases. (6)

"Disappearance Of Glutathione — Glutathione disappears from the lens. (7) In experimentally produced cataract, the freely diffusible cysteine is first changed to its oxidized form and then diffuses out of the lens, whereas the bound cysteine (beta crystallin) is decreased in quantity. (8) It is not known whether the disappearance of glutathione is the cause of cataract formation or whether it is secondary to the cataractous process. As just stated, some evidence exists that the ability of the lens to consume oxygen depends on the presence of glutathione. With the loss of this substance, therefore, the vital power of oxidation of the lens fibers fails. When rats receive galactose, the loss of glutathione precedes the appearance of cataract, and when they are placed back on a normal diet, the glutathione content of the lenses rises so that eventually the rats recover from the incipient cataract. (9) No evidence is available to substantiate this in the case of senile cataract, however, but there is evidence that the experimental cataract due to the administration of naphthalene may be caused by the withdrawal of cystine from the body and consequently from the lens. Naphthalene is detoxificated in the body of the rabbit by conjugation with cysteine and is excreted as alpha-naphthylmercapturic acid. (10) If cystine is given to such experimental animals, the toxicity of naphthalene is reduced and the formation of cataracts is delayed or prevented. (11) No evidence exists that the loss of cysteine or glutathione from the body as a whole or any disturbance in the sulfur metabolism of human beings accounts for senile cataracts. (12) Blood-glutathione determinations done on patients with senile cataracts show no changes from those of normal persons. (13)

"Diminution In Weight — A gradual diminution in the weight of the lens occurs as it becomes cataractous.

27

This is true both of experimental cataract and of ordinary senile cataract. *(14)* By measurement of the slit-lamp optical section, Goldmann *(15)* has demonstrated thinning of the lens in incipient presenile cataract. This change was not defin¹tely found in beginning senile cataract.

"Concentration Of Ascorbic Acid — The concentration of ascorbic acid has been reported to be reduced in the lens. *(16)* What ascorbic acid is present in the aqueous of cataractous eyes is in the oxidized form (dehydro-ascorbic acid) and not in the reduced form as normally occurs. *(17)* However, the loss of ascorbic acid is probably an effect of the cataract rather than the cause of the changes in the lens. It has been suggested that the reduction in the concentration of ascorbic acid in the aqueous in cataract is caused by a reduction in the rate of flow of plasma through the ciliary processes, and experiments indicate that the rate of flow of plasma is less in senile cataract than in eyes with clear lenses. *(18)*

"Some authors believe that the ascorbic acid in the lens remains the same in cataractous lenses as in normal lenses. Purcell and associates *(19)* found the concentration of ascorbic acid in the aqueous to be the same in cataractous eyes as in those with clear lenses.

"Loss Of Protein — A gradual loss of protein, as judged by the nitrogen values in terms of wet weight, occurs in the processes of pathologic sclerosis of the lens and in the formation of cataracts. The average nitrogen content of "practically normal" human lenses is 5.36 percent, decreasing to 4.83 percent during pronounced sclerosis and to 4.43 percent in advanced sclerosis. *(20)* In mature cataracts there is a loss of about 25 percent of the nitrogen. *(21)* The loss is proportional to the degree of damage to the lens and, according to Salit, consists chiefly of the soluble proteins, alpha and beta crystallins. The insoluble albuminoids are left behind and impart increased

28

rigidity and hardness to the nucleus, where they predominate.

"A good deal of interest has centered around changes in blood flow through the ciliary processes and the rate of formation of the aqueous humor in cataractous eyes as compared with normal eyes. While Kronfeld (22) found no change in formation of the aqueous humor in cataractous patients, Linner, (23) using a suction cup method, reports a definite reduction in flow in the presence of cataracts. There was no correlation between the decrease in the rate of flow and the stage of development of the cataract.

REFERENCES

1. Lebensohn, A. E.: Biochemistry of the lens: Mineral metabolism in normal and cataractous lenses, Arch. Ophthal. 15: 217, 1936.

2. Salit, P. W.: The water content and solids of the cataractous and sclerosed human lenses, Amer. J. Ophthal. 21:755, 1938.

3. Salit, P.W., Swan, K.C., and Paul, W.D.: Changes in mineral composition of rat lenses with galactose cataract, Amer. J. Ophthal. 25:1482, 1942.

4. MacKay, G., Stewart, C.P., and Robertson, J.B.: A note on the inorganic constituents of normal and cataractous human crystalline lenses, Brit. J. Ophth. 16:193, 1932.

5. Meesmann, A.: Experimentelle Ultrarotkatarakt durch Langdauernde Schwachdosierte Bestrahlungen Erhielt, Ber. U. Versamml. deutsch. Ophth. Gesellsch. 48:348, 1930.

6. Tsuji, T.: Experimentelle Untersuchungen uber des Linseneiweiss bei Katarakt, J. Biochem. 15:33, 1932.

7. Dische, Z., Borenfreund, E., and Zelmenis, G.: Changes in lens proteins of rats during aging, Arch. Ophthal. 55:471, 1956.

8. Bourne, M.C., and Young, L.: Metabolism of Naphthaline in Rabbits, Biochem. J. 28:803, 1934.

9. Rosner, L., Farmer, C.J., and Bellows, J.: Biochemistry of the lens: Studies on Glutathione in the crystalline lens, Arch. Ophthal, 20:417, 1938.

10. Nakashima, T.: Chemische Untersuchungen uber die Entstehung des Naphthalin — Katarakts, J. Biochem. 19:281, 1934.

11. Bourne, M.C., and Campbell, D.A.: Sulphur metabolism in Senile Cataract, Brit. J. Ophthal. 20:684, 1936.

12. Campbell, D.A.: Glutathione in the blood in Senile Cataract and other ocular conditions. Brit. J. Ophth. 20:33, 1936.

13. Kubik, J.: Sur Pathologic Menschlicher Stare, Arch. Augenheilk. 102:657, 1930.

14. Bellows, J.G.: Biochemistry of the lens: Cevitamic acid content of the blood and urine of subjects with senile cataract, Arch. Ophthal, 15:78, 1936; Some studies on Vitamin C and the lens, Arch. Ophthal. 16:58, 1936.

15. Goldman, H.: Biomicroscopy of the eye, Amer. J. Ophthal. 66:789-804, 1968.

16. Goldmann, H., and Buschke, W.: Blutkammerwasserschranke und Vitamin C; die Permeabilitat der Blutkammerwasserschranke und der Askorbinsaurespiegel der Vorderkammer, Arch. Augenheilk. 109:205, 1935.

17. Day, P.L., Langston, W.C., and O'Brien, C.S.: Cataract and other ocular changes in vitamin G deficiency, Amer. J. Ophthal. 14:1005, 1931.

18. Linner, E.: The rate of plasma flow through the ciliary processes in senile cataract measured by means of ascorbic acid, Acta Ophthal. 32:213, 1954.

19. Purcell, E., Lerner, L., and Kinsey, V.: Ascorbic acid in aqueous

humor and serum of patients with and without cataract, arch. Ophthal. 51:1, 1954.

20. Salit, P.W.: Nitrogen content of cataractous and sclerosed human lenses, Acta Ophthal. 17:81, 1939.

21. Block, R.J., and Salit, P.W.: A note on the amino acids of cataractous and sclerosed human lenses, Arch. Biochem. 10:277, 1946.

22. Kronfeld, P.: Tonography, Arch. Ophthal. 48:393, 1952.

23. Linner, E.: The rate of aqueous flow in human eyes with and without senile cataract, Arch. Ophthal. 61:520, 1959.

4 Causes of Cataract

It appears that all the healing professions disclaim any definite or positive knowledge concerning the cause of senile cataract. I presume they do this because it sort of takes them off the hook. In any event, healers are meant to heal and there is no money in prevention. This I believe is common sense. Now I'm not accusing the healers of withholding any information but basically a healer's work is not prevention. He makes his livelihood by healing. Thus, his forte or general purpose is not giving the cause of the disease or condition. A person does not have to be an Einstein to readily recognize that any condition has to have a cause or contributing factors. It is my sincere and knowledgeable conviction that each and every disease known to man definitely has a cause and when that cause is discovered and removed the condition will cease to exist.

Here in their own words is what the healing professions say concerning the cause of cataract.

''Why cataracts occur is not known, just as we are ignorant of the causes of graying hair or baldness. These phenomena are a part of the ageing process; it has been said that we will all get cataracts if we live long enough (and these days more and more of us live longer)."

"Cataract is a clouding of the lens within the eye. Surgery is the only known effective cure for cataract at present. There is no type of medication that can dissolve a cataract."

I state categorically that many causes of cataract are definitely known. I go further and say that the cause of degenerative or senile cataract is clearly apparent and has been established by medical researchers. Furthermore, protective measures can be followed which will prevent the occurrence of cataract. The medical profession mince no words when they refer to "cures" for cataracts as indicated in the following extract from a medical text — "the only known cure for cataract is surgical removal. No pill, eye drop, injection, or any other substance or procedure will correct or prevent cataracts."

The U.S. Department of Health, Education and Welfare clearly states, "surgery is the only known effective treatment for cataract. Patients should not be misled by the claims of quacks or charlatans that 'magic' salves, drops or pills will dissolve a cataract; it cannot now be done."

I have very thoroughly searched the literature and the records to see if I could find any mention of a positive cause of cataract but nowhere could I find anything specific that was written by the healers. Foremost among the healers is the medical profession. My broad and intensive studies clearly revealed that there are definite causes of cataract. The only reason the medical profession does not know the causes is that they refuse to see. For a medical doctor to say that he does not know the cause of cataract is, in my opinion, an evasion of the truth. Of course he will state that reliable, authentic, medical sources

34

and literature give no cause and therefore he is unable to state the cause of cataract. As I said before, this is a nice easy way for him to get off the hook. To take notice of a non-scientific or a non-medical writer's opinion and findings, no matter how authoritative or well founded, would be absurd and no qualified member of the American Medical Association in good standing would subscribe to that. The medical profession as a body choose to ignore even medical and scientific researchers' findings concerning the cause or causes of cataract.

So here and now I will present what have been found to be the causes of cataract.

FAULTY NUTRITION

It has been proven without a shadow of doubt that nutritional deficiencies are the main cause of cataract where no drug therapy has been used or involved. Medical literature is replete with proof of the fact that vitamin deficiencies are a contributor to, and can cause, cataract. I again must mention that the American Medical Association and most doctors deny that there is a definite cause of cataract or that nutrition could be a factor. Yet clear proof is available in medical literature but 'none are so blind as those who will not see'.

So far in my studies I have found that certain foods have become associated with cataracts and glaucoma. As a matter of fact, there are many clear clues and indications and there appears to be ample evidence to indicate that nutritional factors are mainly involved or responsible. The foremost nutritional factor so far is that various dairy products seem to contribute to cataract. Then it is absolutely clear and scientifically proven that riboflavin or vitamin B2 seems to have an inhibiting or preventive value in cataract.

Recently evidence came to light that indicated that dairy products are probably the leading cause of glaucoma and cataract. I have suspected this for more than 5 years and my suspicions, based on accumulating data, seem to be warranted. In a later chapter I will give you some of the latest evidence.

Back 40 years ago Bernarr Macfadden wrote a book called "Strengthening The Eyes" and here is part of what he had to say about cataracts.

"It is far better to prevent cataracts. This is the sensible approach and can be safely followed with positive assurance that you will not be afflicted with cataract. Also, in their early stages cataracts may frequently be permanently cured. To prevent and cure early stages it is necessary to preserve and restore the general health and learn to use the eyes properly. It is advisable also to follow the suggestions given in this book for eye focusing and eye relaxation.

"Eye-training is of importance in the prevention and the relief of cataract because of the peculiar construction of the lens, and the nature of cataract. The lens is composed of a number of transparent layers lying, like sheets of glass, one upon another. So long as these layers lie flat, light rays pass through them without interference. But when they become warped and more or less separated, as they do in the case of cataract, the lens becomes more or less opaque instead of clear and transparent. A degenerative change takes place in the eye when this condition continues sufficiently long. In this case operation is practically the only means of relief.

"The general state of health has considerable to do with the development of cataract. A state of systemic toxemia, with reduced water content of the blood and with deficient circulation of this nourishing fluid, impairs the nourishment of the lens, causing a dehydration of or loss of water in the lens. This drying out of the lens causes it to become less transparent and more susceptible to derangement by outside pressure of the external eye muscles associated with error of refraction.

"Where there is an incipient cataract it is important that all the laws of health be adhered to. There should be a short fast or fruit diet, with abundant water drinking. The latter diet should be kept down to actual body needs, and it should be highly alkaline in nature. Systemic acidity should be kept down to a minimum. The best alkalinizing foods are the fruits, green and root vegetables and milk — though often it is not advisable for those with developing cataract to drink more than a pint of milk daily. Alcohol, coffee, tea and tobacco should be religiously shunned. Regular exercise of the larger muscles of the body should be taken daily, but there also should be ample relaxation. Daily baths slightly below body temperature, or warm baths followed by cool baths should be taken, followed by good friction. Daily eye-baths such as are advised for congestion of the conjunctiva should be taken daily, and especially the eye relaxation exercises described in these pages under treatment of errors of refraction.

"If these measures are followed from the beginning of any indication of the development of cataract, good results may be expected. Considerable depends, of course, upon the individual's general health and the amount of time given to the treatment, also the mental responsiveness of the patient and the condition of the eye at the time treatment is begun. It is in the initial or functional stages of cataract where best results are obtained. The later stages, those of organic cataract, naturally will make less response. This is true of any organ of the body — functional disorders responding more readily than organic disorders."

The reason that I am quoting Macfadden's writing is

37

to let you see that he did have the approach that something besides surgery was the answer to cataract and that general good health was vitally important.

You will note that back many years Bernarr Macfadden had the gist of the situation as he said, "it is not advisable for those with developing cataract to drink more than a pint of milk daily". This clearly indicates that even 40 years ago there was a suspicion that milk was a factor in cataract. Now I don't know how prevalent pasteurization was then but I know it was done although not as broadly and as widely as it is practiced today and I believe the increase in cataracts is partially due to the heavier indulgence in milk and dairy products as well as to the pasteurization of these products.

Research has indicated that vitamin B2 is essential if cataract is to be prevented. Riboflavin is found abundantly in the retinas of fish eyes. Riboflavin is soluable in water. This means that much of it is lost in cooking. Riboflavin is sensitive to alkali. Riboflavin is sensitive to light. Riboflavin undergoes irreversible decomposition on irradiation with ultra-violet rays or visible light. Riboflavin is reversibly reduced by hydrogen, palladium or platinum and hydrogen, zinc in presence of acid by sodium thiosulfate and by hydrogen sulfide in alkaline solution by titanium chloride. This would lead me to believe that both salt and margarine are positive causes or contributors to cataract and usually margarine contains a lot of salt. So it looks like salt-containing margarine may be one of the big factors in cataract.

It is claimed that at least 90% of the riboflavin in milk is in what is known as a free dialysable form and thus is readily attacked by salt-containing sodium thiosulfate. It is recognized that the sodium thiosulfate in salt is only in minute quantities but obviously it is sufficient to cause the trouble and therefore the greater the intake of salt, the more sodium thiosulfate and the greater the risk of cataract.

Research studies on animals going back more than 40 years have clearly indicated that cataracts will develop in different animals if they are fed a diet deficient in riboflavin. Back in 1931 researchers Day, Langston and O'Brien *(1)* found that 94% of an animal test group fed a diet poor in riboflavin developed cataract in from 60 to 70 days. These findings were confirmed by other researchers on many occasions. A study in 1959 by researchers Gershoff and Andrus discovered bilateral nuclear and subcapsular cataracts in 5 cats fed a high fat, riboflavin deficient diet.

Practically all authorities appear to agree that some constriction of the blood vessels that feed the eye does occur. This selfsame group of blood vessels that feed the eye also in turn remove the wastes. Now we have to decide what causes the constriction. It is generally assumed or recognized that the constriction occurs because of stress or tension felt by the patient, which is passed on to the blood vessels. Here there arises conflicting testimony. It has been recognized that animal fats create a build-up of cholesterol in the walls of the arteries. Could it not be then that this constriction is brought about by a narrowing of the arterial walls due to a build-up of cholesterol?

So here we have to decide what brings on the constriction . . . stress and tension or a build-up of cholesterol in the arterial walls or deficient nutrition which fails to nourish and sustain the elasticity or integrity of the blood vessels. As the build-up increases the passage way for the blood becomes narrower and narrower so that the eye becomes starved for the cellular regenerative nutrients. Back before the 1840's it was stated that people under 40 never had cataracts. Statistics clearly indicate that cataract cases have been rising steadily for the past twenty or so years since records of cataract surgery are available. It is also of interest to note that atherosclerosis or heart disease has also increased greatly as has the use of animal fats such as meat, butter, cream, cheese and eggs, all of which contribute to cholesterol build-up in the arteries. It is my opinion and feeling that the cholesterol is definitely a factor in cataract. I do not entirely dismiss stress as a factor but I feel that the stress is caused or accentuated by the cholesterol build-up which narrows the opening through which the blood runs.

Dr. Harry Eggers, director of Ophthalmology, St. Luke's Hospital, New York, in the pages of the Journal of the American Geriatric Society for May, 1966 mentions that he sees many elderly patients daily who are blind or partially blind, because the arteries of the eye have been disabled by the process of atherosclerosis, which we call 'hardening'. It is a process in which fatty substances like cholesterol are deposited on the inside of the artery, narrowing it, so that blood cannot get through in sufficient quantity.

Dr. Eggers goes on to state that "It can be prevented and it can even be stopped once it has started. Except for those people who have an inherited defect which early in life disordered the way their bodies used fatty substances, one can control the situation chiefly by limiting his intake of so-called saturated fats and increasing his intake of unsaturated fats."

Then Dr. Eggers gives very simple directions for planning diets along these lines and points out the places where most of us make our biggest mistake in diet. The fats that should be greatly reduced in the diet are: meat fats, milk fats, hydrogenated vegetable oils (creamy shortenings and commerical margarines), coconut oil, palm oil and chocolate. Meat fats mean all visible fat in the meat, bacon and processed products such as sausage, salami, bologna, frankfurter and liverwurst. Gravy is forbidden unless it is first defatted by chilling and skimming off all visible fat. Hamburgers should be avoided unless they are prepared at home from lean meats. Milk fats mean whole milk, butter, cream, ice cream and all cheeses except those made from skim milk. Hydrogenated margarine and shortening are just as harmful or even more harmful than lard or butter. Bakery products made with lard, coconut oil, palm oil, butter, cream or hydrogenated vegetable oil should be avoided.

There you have it. It would appear as though the animal fats are a factor in contributing to cataract.

There is evidence that the improper use or assimilation of calcium is a contributing factor in cataract. This has another link. In a test on mice where they were fed on yogurt, 100% of the mice in the experiment developed cataract in short order. Now this was commercial yogurt and invariably it is made with pasteurized milk. It is established that in the process of pasteurization or when calcium is not balanced by phosporus, due to lack of magnesium it becomes difficult or impossible for the body to assimilate calcium properly. Thus the body deposits the calcium or some of the calcium on the lens of the eye.

Dr. A. Cantarow also claims that lack of calcium allows cataracts to form. I presume he means assimilable calcium. It is also known that vitamin C is absolutely essential to help calcium function properly.

Researchers working on the Etiology of Senile Cataract learned that there was a marked change in the protein content of the lens when it was affected with cataract. The normal lens, it is claimed, contains approximately 35% soluble or organic protein, whereas the lens that shows advanced opacity contains greater amounts of insoluble protein and smaller amounts of soluble protein.

41

It is clear that a shifting balance in the levels of the soluble and insoluble protein takes place in the senile cataract lens where the soluble protein diminishes more rapidly than the insoluble protein. So there we have it. There is not only a change in the type of protein but a natural loss in the total amount of protein as well. So it is obvious from this research project that the eye, when it is affected by cataract, appears to be improperly or inadequately nourished.

Another important change was noticed in the advanced senile opacity and that was the lowering of the amount of water in the lens. That is, the lens of advanced cataract appeared to be dry. It was also found that there was a reduced amount of vitamin C in the cataract-affected lens.

One must not jump to the conclusion that vitamin C is the big or important factor in cataract because research does not indicate this to be true. Researchers increased considerably the amount of vitamin C in the diets of people with cataract with little or no effect. However, when riboflavin and vitamin C are administered together the increase in the vitamin C level of the eye is most marked.

I would like to point out at this time that this indicates the importance in the diet of greens and grains together because the greens will give you all the vitamin A and C plus others and the grains will give you all the B vitamins plus others including riboflavin. Now you see why I stress the importance of foods rich in vitamins A, B2 and C as among the essential foods for good eye health.

From some of the statistics that I was able to obtain it appears that in 1963 there were 200,000 cataract operations in the United States. In 1970 this figure rose to 400,000. I'm suggesting now in 1973-74 that the figure is closer to 500,000.

Without trying to read into the record something that does not exist I'd like to bring to your attention something which maybe has greater importance than appears on the surface.

Remember, cataracts have more than doubled, in fact increased two and a half times, in the past 10 years. Margarine has only come into its own in the past 10 or 15 years. Could widespread use of margarine be a factor in cataracts and other eye disorders? Yes, even in cataracts in youth or congenital cataract. Butter as we know it, good wholesome butter, contains some vitamin B2 and C and adequate or large quantities of vitamins A and D. I'm suggesting that margarine contains little if any vitamin B2 or C. I know that margarine contains lots of A and D because it is added . . . but synthetically. Therefore, I'm suggesting that the body can absorb and utilize vitamins A, B2, C and D but when these vitamins are synthesized and added to margarine the body can only metabolize minute quantities and thus the eye conditions are created because of a deficiency of these essential vitamins.

Please do not ignore this theory.

Here is another reference which indicates that the medical fraternity claims that the cause of cataracts are unknown. "The type of cataract that occurs in elderly people known as senile cataract has no known etiology."

From Adler's Physiology Of The Eye we learn, "Galactose and Xylose Cataracts — The presence of high levels of d-galactose or d-xylose in the aqueous inevitably leads to the formation of cataract. Galactose cataract can be produced experimentally by feeding a diet containing more than 25 percent galactose. Galactose also occurs in a rare inborn error of metabolism in human infants known as

43

galactosemia in which the infant is unable to metabolize one of the components of lactose (galactose). This is due to the deficiency of an enzyme, galactose 1-phosphate uridyl transferase, necessary for the conversion of galactose to glucose.

"As a result of this metabolic block, galactose and galactose 1-phosphate accumulate in the blood and in the aqueous. Infants with this deficiency are normal at birth but soon feeding becomes a problem and they fail to thrive. Cataracts begin to appear very early in over half the patients. If the disease is detected early, and if all milk and other foods containing lactose or galactose are eliminated from the diet, recovery may be rapid and the lens opacities may disappear."

Here in the one column on the one page they say that senile cataract has no known etiology and here right beside it on the same page they tell you one cause of cataract.

"Amino acid deficiency cataracts. Diets deficient in protein, especially proteins containing tryptophan, will produce cataracts in young guinea pigs. (2) Unlike most forms of experimental cataract studied, the changes in the lens in this type of cataract are not found at the lens equator, all components of which retain their normal appearance, but at the ends of the lens fibers, particularly at the suture lines. A diet deficient in many other amino acids has likewise been found to be cataractogenic. This is particularly true of diets deficient in phenylalanine, valine, and histidine. (3) Cataract formation caused by such dietary deficiencies has never been noted in human infants."

It has been found that diarrhea, vomiting, ulcers, hyperthyroidism and various other infections tend to waste or lose riboflavin. They are supposed to be recognized as positive riboflavin antagonists and wasters. I'm suggesting that there are other things that waste the riboflavin and among them are coffee, tea, alcohol, soft drinks, chlorine, fluorine and tobacco.

Research indicates that deficiencies of vitamin B6 (pyridoxine) and tryptophane, which is one of the amino acids, are known to be a contributing factor in cataract.

Dr. Donald Gustofson and co-workers have stated in an article "Malnutrition as an Etiological (Causative) Factor in Senile Cataract" claims there has been a great deal of professional debate about the possibility of cataract resulting from dehydration of the lens — that is, perhaps the water was extracted from it. Cholera patients, it seems, go blind in the last stages of their illness because the lenses of their eyes dry out.

LACK OF VITAMIN D AND SUNLIGHT

Seldom, if ever, is it mentioned that vitamin D could be a factor in disorders of the eyes. I made a careful study of the various effects of vitamin D deficiency and somehow I have the feeling, if not conclusive proof, that vitamin D is a factor in conditions involving the eyes such as cataract and glaucoma.

You must understand that sunlight does play a vital part in our health and welfare. I wouldn't suggest that you would die quickly or suffer any tremendous amount of disease if you didn't get a fair amount of sunlight because there happen to be many occupations that deny a man much sunlight. However, it must be admitted that sunlight is not only important but vital in the maintenance of all-round good health of a human being.

As most of the people of America live in the temperate zone we must deal with that area. Shackleton, the world famous explorer who spent a long time in the polar areas stated "At the close of the night of four months' duration our faces were greenish yellow, but the sun soon tanned us again. Yet stranger was the discovery that the eyes of almost all of those which were brown and black became blue or gray during the long night."

William J. Fielding in his book "The Marvels and Oddities of Sunlight" quotes Widmer "The skin of the parts of the body exposed to the light shows a tremendous increase in 'turgor'. After a short time it becomes 'full' and padded out, and wrinkles and corners are smoothed away. The whole individual is beautified," he writes, and this observation has been confirmed by others with sufficient experience in sunlight therapy to speak with authority.

Let us note that from November til March the hours of sunlight are greatly reduced. The longest day, as we know, is June 22nd and the shortest day is December 22nd. Studies reveal that when there is inadequate sunlight — that is, short days and long nights and also when people are inclined to stay indoors the eyes have been found to contain approximately one third of the quantity of vitamin D compared to what they contain during optimum sunlight. This was proved by the famed team of medical researchers, Bicknell and Prescott.

Furthermore, the milk, butter and eggs that are consumed in the winter contain less than one third of the normal vitamin D.

During the winter many people do not eat nearly the amount of vegetables that they do in the summer. Many people have gardens and they get their vegetables from their gardens along with the vitamin D from the sun and atmosphere in the summer.

"Cataract, according to Maxwell and Pi, (4) is found in at least fifteen percent of marked cases of osteomalacia.

46

The condition develops slowly, and in its early stages can only be diagnosed with a slit lamp. It is important to consider whether cataract in young and middle-aged women may not be caused by undiagnosed osteomalacia which is still only causing vague pain in the back and limbs. Treatment of the underlying deficiency of vitamin D may improve the cataract."

"In myopia and trachoma no results have been obtained with vitamin D given by mouth, while in iritis and conjunctivitis injections of vitamins A and D are said to be of value, and so is cod liver oil applied to the eye in phlyctenular conjunctivitis. (5) The improvement in the latter two conditions was probably caused by vitamin A. Keratoconus has been reported to improve with calcium and vitamin D. There is no confirmation of the experimental and clinical work of Knapp that lack of vitamin D causes retinitis pigmentosa in the dog and that in man this condition, myopia and night blindness are improved by vitamin D and calcium."

I believe that vitamin D is an important factor and anyone who is suffering from eye conditions would be well advised to insure a supply of assimilable vitamin D from some of the foods that I have mentioned plus the best form of vitamin D that is available by exposure to the outdoors and sunlight.

Research indicates that vitamin D deficiency is definitely involved in the formation of cataracts, mainly because of its effect on calcium metabolism.

A researcher by the name of Goldmann did a very thorough study in which he induced periods of tetany in dogs by withholding calcium in the diet. When he did this he produced subcapsular opacities during the period of calcium deprivation. In the intervening tetany free periods new clear fibers were laid down in the lens. By repeating

47

the process frequently researcher Goldmann was able to observe alternating layers of opaque and clear lens fibers, indicating an obvious relationship between the subcapsular cataract and the calcium deficiency of tetany. Researchers Swan and Salet created cataracts in 49 rabbits which were maintained on a low calcium diet. It has long been established that vitamin D is essential for proper calcium metabolization.

It has definitely been established that a calcium build-up is associated with cataract. Here it is learned that cataract is caused by calcium deprivation. Contradictory, no? However, I have clearly pointed out that the body can only properly metabolize calcium in its natural form as found in uncooked, untreated foods or unpasteurized milk or unprocessed dairy foods. Further, in raw natural foods the calcium is found with practically all other vitamins and minerals and a full quota of active enzymes.

While there are people who are affected with conditions or diseases known as light sensitivity, meaning they can't stand very much sunlight, in general more people suffer injury because of lack of sunlight. Such conditions are known as sensitizer illnesses.

The human body has been so constructed that it is intended that the amount of vitamin D required would be derived from the action of the sun and the atmosphere upon the skin but because we are practically covered with clothes from top to bottom this means that the body receives a minimal amount of sunlight. In fact, sometimes it is almost totally absent.

A further point must be mentioned and that is that by the use of soaps and detergents the ability of the skin to absorb vitamin D from sunlight and the atmosphere is impaired. Because everybody uses soap the average body is sorely deficient in vitamin D.

The body is made up and functions by means of all nutrients and elements and vitamins. Therefore, if one specific vitamin is absent or in minimal supply this can contribute to various conditions and diseases. I further suggest that vitamin D from unnatural or synthetic sources, such as vitamin supplement pills, is poorly absorbed or metabolized, if it can be metabolized at all, by the body. Granted, there are some foods that contain vitamin D but again it is a question as to whether or not the body can properly utilize and assimilate that vitamin D. I still have the feeling that nature intended that vitamin D be derived from the sun and the atmosphere and their action upon the human body.

In our modern industrial age the smoke, smog and other pollutants in the air are a factor in preventing the proper absorption of various elements from the atmosphere. Thus I'm suggesting that the human body is suffering from sunlight starvation. It is a statistical fact that older people tend to die in greater numbers towards the end of the winter and just before spring makes its appearance. Here I'm suggesting that there may be a relationship in the amount of vitamin D and as the amount drops below a certain level, death occurs. This is not directly because of lack of vitamin D but because the body cannot utilize the other vitamins due to insufficient vitamin D.

I'd like to quote something by C. W. Saleeby, a British medical writer. In referring to the skin he stated, "This admirable organ, the natural clothing of the body, which grows continuously throughout life, which has at least four absolutely distinct sets of sensory nerves distributed to it, which is essential in the regulation of the temperature, which is waterproof from without inwards, but allows the excretory sweat to escape freely, which, when unbroken, is microbe-proof, and which can readily absorb sunlight — this most beautiful, versatile and wonderful organ is, for the most part, smothered, blanched

49

and blinded in clothes, and can only gradually be restored to the air and light which are its natural surroundings. Then, and only then, we learn what it is capable of."

From the evidence I have presented I want to make it clear that I feel the lack of sunlight, especially directly to the eyes, is a factor in cataract, glaucoma and perhaps other eye disorders.

STRESS AND STRAIN

Many authorities contend that tension and stress are big factors in cataract. I feel that when the body is properly nourished stress is not a factor. But most people do not have a proper diet and thus 'stress' is a factor. Among the stress factors are the following: fears, resentments, vehement hatred, worries, occupational pressures and accidents.

This may sound contradictory because some experts clearly contend that stress constricts some of the muscles and they are the arterial system that feeds the eyes. This causes or contributes to cataract. It is of great importance that you know and understand that a healthy person in good physical condition does not have cataracts nor does his body develop cataracts unless through accident or due to congenital abnormalities. Therefore, if you follow a correct pattern of living and eating you will never develop cataracts. This does not imply or suggest that you can maintain or continue your present way of life because you think it is right and thus avoid cataracts because that may be far from the truth. At 30, 40 or even at 50 years of age sometimes we think we are in perfect health and we think we are doing what is right and we think we are eating properly.

Here I am stressing that thinking is not enough. You must be sure that you are getting proper nourishment and

50

that you are in healthy condition and there is not much use running to your doctor to find out whether or not you are healthy because healthy people don't go to doctors and most doctors wouldn't know a healthy person if they fell over one. I'm not trying to be funny and I'm not casting reflections . . . I'm telling an honest straight-forward truth. There is not much sense in going to a doctor and asking him for a diet sheet or asking him for instructions regarding food and nutrition because few, if any, doctors in America have studied nutrition. Then those few who did study nutrition studied it on the basis of what the food processors, the chemical corporations, the National Academy of Sciences, the National Research Council taught them. Let me strongly assert that the courses they teach and the texts and information they provide are based upon the recommendations of all of the bodies that I mentioned who are not concerned about your health but only concerned about selling you counterfeit foods and drugs and these are the people who teach the medical profession the little bit they know about nutrition. So don't go to a doctor looking for information concerning your nutritional problems because he can't help you.

It is also essential that you know that the National Research Council and the National Academy of Sciences are not unbiased, unprejudiced, scientific bodies. These authoritative-sounding, scientific organizations are in absolute truth only so-called scientific branches of the food processors, beverage makers and the chemical and drug corporations. If you doubt me, write to the National Research Council or the National Academy of Sciences at Independence Square, Washington, D.C. and ask them.

In spite of the fact that practically all authorities on the eyes, including ophthalmologists, warn against straining the eyes or using them too much and causing injury, it is my belief . . . and I've said so on many occasions . . . that using the eyes even under stress is not seriously harmful.

Recently — in 1972 — the Illinois society for the Prevention of Blindness went on record as stating that you cannot possibly injure the eyes by using them too much. Yes, your eyes may feel tired, they may ache or feel heavy or maybe your sight is diminished for a period but that does not contribute to their deterioration. Their findings stated that they may be used during the entire waking day without any resulting harm. They further stated that if one is reading in poor light or is out on the beach in the sunshine and there is a great deal of glare one may experience discomfort and temporary inconvenience.

In a report from the British Medical Journal for August 15th, 1953, Dr. J. H. Doggert says "It is almost impossible to damage the eyes by long hours of reading and sewing, even if great fatigue is experienced at the time."

I have maintained for years that the used muscle is a strong muscle and the more you use your eyes in more varied positions and views the stronger and healthier they will be. I have known people who read long hours under poor light and they did not suffer any injury. Where there is a great deal of glare I would suggest protecting the eyes by shading them. Hard usage will not harm the eyes but using them improperly or applying treatments of any kind can cause harm.

According to some eminent medical authorities the lens is the weak link in the body chain. I might say that with this opinion I strongly disagree.

DRUGS

Some drugs are known to cause cataract, especially the corticosteroids such as cortisone. Medical literature is full of cases where cataract appeared after the use of cortisone or other corticosteroids. If you have taken or used cortisone or other corticosteroid drugs there is grave danger of cataract developing. Steroid therapy is positively linked in the cause of cataracts.

Here we have some information concerning corticosteroid treatment.

"Cataracts are a well described complication of long-term corticosteroid treatment. This complication is known to occur mainly in patients who have received corticosteroid therapy for more than two years. In one study cataracts appeared in patients who had received prednisone for an average period of 3-7 years, whereas no cataracts were noted in patients treated with corticosteroids for less than a year.

"Posterior subcapsular cataracts occurred in four children who had received corticosteroid therapy for periods ranging from three to 10 months. Two children had systemic lupus erythematosus complicated by nephritis; one had juvenile rheumatoid arthritis, and one Takayasu's disease. The range of prednisone dosage varied from 1 to 3 mg. per kilogram of body weight in two cases, and the equivalent dose of paramethasone in the other cases. Cataracts were discovered after careful and repeated ophthalmologic examination with the slit lamp.

"Our findings seem to disagree with the opinion of some authors who suggest that cataracts appear only after prolonged treatment with corticosteroids, and seem to favour the opinion of others who relate the presence of cataracts not only to duration and dose of corticosteroid treatment but also to individual susceptibility. It is interesting that two of the patients included in the study carried out in India had cataracts within a year of receiving therapy with corticosteroids. Our four Mexican cases as well as those reported from India seem to suggest not only an individual susceptibility but also a susceptibility based on genetic differences due to a different ethnic origin." (6)

Dimethyl sulfoxide which was so highly recommended and touted by the medical and drug fraternities as being a miracle drug has been shown and proven to contribute to or cause cataract. Evidently, before DMSO really got off the ground, in spite of the good press, it was found to cause many serious conditions and the drug corporations and the medical profession dropped it like a hot potato. Evidently the damage it caused was much too great and the results were too quick in appearing for either the medical profession or the drug corporations to keep it around . . . so they buried it. I distinctly recall reading a tremendous amount of literature boosting DMSO when this drug first was introduced.

Dimethyl sulfoxide is used as a solvent for acetylene, sulfur dioxide and other gases. As antifreeze or hydraulic fluid when mixed with water. Solvent for Orlon. As paint and varnish remover. Dissolves some hydrocarbons more than others. We find this information in the Merck Index, seventh edition.

Tranquilizers are definitely established as being a cause of cataract. "M. Varga and P. Jabbagy, ophthalmologists from Hungary have reported cases of cataract associated with the use of tranquilizer therapy. In this specific instance the drug Quietidin, which is a piperazine derivative, was the culprit. The reports concerned ten patients who developed photodermatitis and then cataract in the posterior lens cortex. Stopping the medication checked progression of both conditions. Other Hungarian doctors have found similar consequences. One of these suggests that decomposition of the drug may upset the chemical balance of the organism, as a result of which there may be a breakdown in resistance to detrimental or excessive exposure to light.

"Intensive research is recommended on the incidence of cataract development following excessive administration of tranquilizing drugs. We suggest discontinuing the use of the drug."

The following is further proof concerning tranquilizers and cataract.

"Tranquilizers May Be Hazardous To Eyes — Potent tranquilizing drugs employed effectively in mental hospitals constitute a two-edged medical tool, presenting a hazard of serious eye defects for a significant proportion of patients, a New York eye specialist said recently.

"Dr. Irving H. Leopold of Mt. Sinai Hospital said cataracts, clouding of the cornea, and degeneration of the retina are not uncommon adverse side effects of the use of such drugs in the large doses over extended periods of time required for treating the severely mentally ill.

"He said such effects can begin after about seven or eight years' use of the drugs in those patients who, for reasons still unknown, are genetically vulnerable to such adverse side effects." (7)

Dinitrophenol was one of the first to attract attention because of the high incidence of cataracts in human beings taking this drug for obesity. The drug busulfan (Myleran), used in the treatment of myeloid leukemia, has likewise been found to be cataractogenic in rats, and recently triparanol (Mer/29), used for the control of hypercholesteremia, has definitely produced cataracts in human beings and has now been withdrawn from the market. We must be constantly on the alert for such untoward side effects when new drugs are prescribed.

Cataracts have been produced experimentally by the introduction of many different toxic substances, either fed or injected, such as naphthalene, mimosene, and quinoid substances.

Cataracts have been known to occur in individuals exposed to intense radiation. Microwaves have produced cataracts in rabbits. *(8)*

It must be recognized that many drugs, shots, injections, even those used for protective measures or used in immunization for smallpox, diphtheria, measles, chickenpox, whooping cough may contribute to eye problems and affect vision. This is especially true when these substances are taken by or injected into a pregnant woman because frequently they affect the unborn and result in various birth defects and some of these include the eye.

The most serious and disquieting factor about the effects of drugs on the eyes is the fact that in practically every instance the damage done to the eyes is irreversible, even when the drug use and treatment have stopped.

SUGAR

I consider sugar to be a causative factor in one or many ways. Perhaps it, too, is antagonistic or destructive of various vitamins essential for the eyes. Then perhaps sugar leaches out or wastes essential nutrients to an alarming degree. It is my belief that it is worse than anyone suspects or realizes. However, this has not as yet been scientifically established.

A report that appeared in the Nutrition Review of Sept. 1965 tells us cataracts were developed experimentally in rats which were made diabetic or hypergalactosemic (suffering from excess milk-sugar) by feeding them diets higher in sugar alcohols such as sorbitol and dulcitol. (These are chemical forms of sugar. Some are from basic natural sources, but by no means any longer natural.)

Now I quote from the Textbook of Biochemistry,

page 1176. "Lactose: The digestion products of lactose are glucose and galactose. The liver converts galactose to glucose. Lactose provides the total carbohydrate intake of infants and animals ingesting only milk. This attests to the nutritive value of the sugar (lactose).

"Certain unexplained findings in regard to the experimental feeding of lactose or of galactose are of interest. It has been known for some time that feeding rats diets high in lactose *(9)* or galactose *(10)* leads to the development of a type of cataract. Day *(11)* amply confirmed these observations and also determined blood sugar in rats eating diets containing 60% of various carbohydrates . . .

"Of 18 rats on the lactose ration, 17 developed cataract at an average time of 44 days. Three rats given the galactose ration showed cataracts on the 11th day. None of the animals eating the rations containing sucrose, glucose, or starch showed cataracts. The cataracts were said to be readily distinguishable from the cataracts that develop in rats as a result of riboflavin deficiency. The relationship between the incidence of cataract and high blood sugar is not clear. In diabetes mellitus the incidence of cataract is apparently higher than in the healthy individual.

"The poor nutritive value of lactose when it constitutes the sole carbohydrate of rations of animals past the weaning age is attested to by many reports. Growth of such animals is invariably poorer with this sugar constituting the dietary carbohydrate than when sucrose, glucose, or starch is employed."

'With animals long-continued and well-controlled deficiency experiments are practical. Rats exhibit decreased growth rate, eye changes, including a keratitis and rather typical cataracts, dermatitis, possibly a type of anemia, some nerve degeneration, and poor reproduction.

57

Congenital malformation *(12)* and cessation of the estrous cycle *(13)* have been reported. Definite symptoms of ariboflavinosis in calves have been reported. *(14)"*

"Galactoflavin is a potent riboflavin antagonist. Emerson and co-workers *(15)* reported marked growth inhibitions in rats on diets containing this compound. The effect was found to be largely removed by the addition to the diet of sufficient riboflavin."

THE ROLE OF SODIUM NITRATE AND NITRITE IN CATARACT

In a report from Rome it appears that certain wines have been known to cause blindness. The wine which was said to be produced for domestic consumption had been treated with sodium nitrate to prevent quick fermentation. Eighteen wine-makers in a renowned grape-growing area of the Alban Hills in Italy have been charged with having adulterated their wine with toxic substances. Their names were deliberately withheld. Obviously sodium nitrate can cause or contribute to cataract and blindness. Remember, sodium nitrate is widely used in meats as a means of maintaining color and also to prevent spoilage of the meat. Luncheon meats, cured meats, hot dogs, corned beef and practically all meats but fresh meats are loaded with sodium nitrate and nitrite and this includes bacon. So I'm sure that the American public gets more than a fair share of the ubiquitous sodium nitrate. Thus I warn . . . don't eat meats or any other food that contains sodium nitrate or nitrite.

OTHER CONTRIBUTING FACTORS

Medical records show that cataracts and other defects may occur in certain infants whose mothers had German measles early in their pregnancies; such cataracts can be prevented by protecting the mothers from exposure to measles during the early months of pregnancy or as suggested by the medical fraternity, exposing girls to German measles before their child-bearing years.

Just what part smog and polluted air play in cataract has not been established but no one would dare rule out smog and pollution as contributing factors in cataract.

My personal experience with smog and air pollution clearly indicates that there is a link with eye troubles. I have undergone severe physical pain and distress because of smog and pollution and it seriously affected both my vision and my perceptibility, apart from the severe pain.

The use of laxatives or mineral oils which usually contain liquid paraffin definitely decrease or prevent the proper absorption of vitamins A, D, E and K and therefore the use of laxatives containing mineral oil or paraffin is definitely linked as a cause of cataract.

Salt may be a factor in cataracts. Dr. Donald T. Atkinson in his article "Malnutrition as an Etiological (Causative) Factor in Senile Cataract" mentions an experiment in which a frog placed in salt water soon develops cataract because the salt affects the water in the lens of the eye. Then if the frog is put back into fresh water the cataract disappears. Now it all depends on your viewpoint. I suggest this indicates that a heavy salt intake might or could be a factor in cataract.

Fluorescent and ultraviolet light are recognized as contributors to cataract. Also, glaring light. Long hours of television watching, especially colored television, is linked as a causative factor. It is known that the big picture tube is radioactive and, as we know that fluorescent light and ultraviolet light destroy vitamin B2, the connection is cemented. It is recommended that when you watch television you stay 6 feet at least from the black and white and 12 feet at least from colored television. One authority suggested to me that this distance should be doubled to be sure of minimizing the effects of radiation.

In cases where children or young people have cataracts and where it is definitely not due to congenital circumstances I'm suggesting it is due to the care given by the mother or the nurse, whichever the case may be. Today infants and children are washed a great deal with strong soaps and they are also given various drugs; for example, the hexachloraphene that was so widely used in practically every hospital in the world. I claim that hexachloraphene and strong soaps and other drugs are the basic cause of cataract in children and young people.

One of the basic reasons for this is the prevention of the absorption of vitamin D by the infant or child and, since they are deficient in vitamin D, there we have the firm basis for the cause of cataract because with no vitamin D the other essential vitamins are handicapped and do not function properly. Without a supply of vitamin D the cataract build-up commences. Therefore, I strongly suggest a deficiency of vitamin D caused by the excessive use of soaps and drugs is a very vital factor in cataracts in young people. Do not compare senile or degenerative cataract with congenital or drug induced cataracts.

I have stumbled upon an interesting and perhaps an enlightening bit of information concerning a causative factor in cataract and this might well be the most important piece of information in this book. As I have stated throughout the book, eye glasses or contact lens are in no way beneficial to the condition of the eyes. In no way do they improve anything pertaining to the eyes. They do magnify the object that you are looking at and thus make it easier to see but they in no way contribute any benefit whatsoever to the eyes. On the other hand it is a known fact that they do contribute harm to varying degrees from a little bit of harm to a great deal of harm.

Now comes the crux. Recent studies indicate that glasses and probably contact lenses are contributing factors if not definitely causative factors in cataracts. Furthermore, the reasons for this condition or the proof is not difficult to come by or understand. It has been explained elsewhere in this book the eyes are not supplied with the same blood vessel system as other parts of the body and the reason is clear and simple. If the eyes were completely laced with blood vessels it would interfere with light passing through the lens or the cornea. Nature had to devise a different method of supplying nutrients and removing waste from the eyes. Therefore, the system that nature provided or devised is intricate and can be more easily damaged, injured or harmed than other parts of the body.

I'm sure that every human being has long learned that the eyes are a very, very sensitive part of the anatomy and, as you may well understand, nature never intended that the eyes would be covered with magnifying glasses to improve vision. So this was not taken into consideration when nature created the eyes and the food supplying and drainage system. O.K., now we have it. We take a normal pair of eyes and we put glasses on them. Immediately the metabolism, the functioning, the workings are slowed down because the eye no longer has to work in order to see clearly, because of the magnification. Thus, slowly but positively stagnation results and this could actually be the beginning and the cause of cataract. The aqueous solution becomes impaired because the muscles all become weak from the lack of exercise or functioning ability with consequent weakening of constricting and expansion ability and cannot supply the essential nutrients. This in the long run causes malnutrition in the eye and we have the beginning of cataract. It has been established that people who have long worn glasses are the first victims of cataract.

61

The more I study, the more I read, the more I observe concerning cataract and glaucoma the more it becomes clear and apparent that the causes of both conditions are similar, almost to the point of being identical. Basically, it is the inability of the eye to feed and drain itself. The way I look at it today is that in cataract the eye is poorly nourished. The supply route is bad or failing and the eye is thus grossly undernourished.

In glaucoma, evidently the food supply channels are more open but the drainage channels are inadequate for the amount of nutrients that are supplied and this creates a build-up and tremendous pressure in the eyes and this brings about severe pain.

So in one case we have an inadequate food supply and normal or slow drainage whereas in the other case we have a greater food supply but totally inadequate drainage. This appears to me to be the principle difference between cataract and glaucoma.

It is stated that because the lens is an organ which does not possess any blood vessels no inflammation or inflammatory processes can occur. It is claimed that this is the reason why degenerative conditions set in and frequently progress rapidly and this leads to cloudiness of the lens tissue and the development of cataract.

Here is what one authority claims are the four factors which contribute to the loss of transparency of the lens substance and thus to the weakening of sight. 1) Stagnation of the fluid current in the lens resulting from a blood condition. 2) Deterioration in the nutrition of the lens which diminishes the vitality and resistance of the delicate lens fibers. 3) Deposits between the lens fibers of acids and salts which have an irritating effect on the lens tissue and exert an increasing pressure on its delicate fibers, gradually destroying them. 4) Unless appropriate measures are taken in time the lens fibers finally disintegrate and break down and the whole lens becomes clouded.

Something that has puzzled me for many years is that many people claim horses suffer from cataracts. I have given this matter considerable study and attention and eventually I struck upon what I believe to be the answer. At the present time horses are not used very much on farms but there are many horses used on the racetracks and in the western States and also the western part of Canada horses are still used for riding or for the showring. Well, why would horses be subject to cataract? I think I can give you the reason.

Their food is no longer the food they would get if they were on a regular farm. That is, grass and some grains. Yes, they still get grass, grass from heavily fertilized fields loaded with nitrogen and other chemicals and grains that have been broken up or chopped with various chemicals added to prevent or to try to prevent the grains from becoming rancid. Also, most of the manufactured feeds are composed of residues and wastes from sugar manufacture, oil extraction and other such sources. It is my sincere belief that the loss of the vital elements, minerals and vitamins from the chopping of these grains is the main contributing factor in creating cataract in the horses. I would be willing to wager $1,000 that if horses were fed good hay and whole grains, oats preferably, there would be no cataract nor any other disease.

From the information that I have accumulated it would appear that the eyes are the mirror of what goes on inside your body. They are actually an indication of the health level of the entire body. It appears that even the slightest disorder inside is expressed in your eyes. Or put it this way . . . when your eyes are sound and healthy your body is sound and healthy. One must judge somewhat by one's personal experiences and I have found that when I'm

63

not in top form my eyes seem to express it.

REFERENCES

1. Day, P.L., Langston, W.C., and O'Brien, C.S., "Cataract and other ocular changes in vitamin G Deficiency." Am. J. Ophth., 1931, 14, 1005.

2. Von Sallmann, L., Reid, M., Grimes, P., and Collins, E.: Tryptophan-deficiency cataract in guinea pigs, Arch. Ophthal. 62:662, 1959.

3. Hall, W., Bowles, I., Sydenstricker, V., and Schmidt, H.: Cataracts due to deficiencies of phenylalanine and histidine in the rat: a comparison with other types of cataract, J. Nutrition 36:277, 1948.

4. Maxwell, J.P., and Pi, H.T. "Cataract in Adult Rickets (Osteomalacia)." Proc. Roy. Soc. Med., 1940, 33, 777.

5. Cameron, A.J. "Cod Liver Oil In External Eye Affections". B. M. J., 1936, ii., 785.

6. The New England Jn. Of Med., 280:3. '72-160. Quoted from Bombay Indian Med. Assoc., Vol. 1:3 — July, 1972.

7. National Health Federation Bulletin, January, 1966.

8. Williams, D., Monohan, J., Nicholson, W., and Aldrich, J.: Biologic effects studies on microwave radiation, Arch. Ophthal. 54:863, 1955.

9. Mitchell, H.S., J. Nutrition, 9, 37, 1935.

10. Mitchell, H.S., Proc. Soc. Exptl. Biol. Med., 32, 971, 1935.

11. Day, P.L., J. Nutrition, 12, 395, 1936.

12. Warkany, J., and Schraffenberger, E., J. Nutrition, **27**, **477**, 1944.

13. Coward, K.H., and Morgan, B.G.E., Biochem. J., 35, 974, 1941.

14. Wiese, A.C., Johnson, B.C., Mitchell, H.H., and Nevens, W.B., J. Nutrition, 33, 263, 1947.

15. Emerson, G.A., Wurtz, E., and Johnson, J.H., J. Biol. chem., 160, 165, 1945.

5 Milk, Milk Products and Cataract

I make no apologies for stating that I believe the use of dairy products to be a factor in cataract. Let it be understood that I feel quite certain that there are people who never drank a drop of milk or used any dairy products who have had cataracts. This does not alter the fact that I believe dairy products can be and are a factor in the development and creation of cataracts in the human eye.

In fairness to milk and dairy products I want it stated and clearly understood that I am not blaming or condemning milk per se but I am asking you to consider (1) pasteurization, (2) the various, many and devious processes and treatments, (3) the many antibiotics, drugs and chemical treatments that are given the cows and the milk and the milk containers. The whole, unpasteurized milk itself could be totally and completely innocent but with this series of involvements I suggest therein lies the cause for it being a contributing factor in the causation of cataract. Therefore, beware of milk and dairy products in any form, especially if they form a major portion of your diet.

It came as no surprise to me when a friend of mine developed serious troubles with his eyes and became temporarily blind and eventually lost the total sight of one eye. He was not a milk user but he did love his cheese. He could eat half a pound or even a pound of cheese at a sitting and all of his friends knew his weakness for cheese. Apart from the cheese he lived a rather simple existence and watched his foods and followed the "hygienist" way of living. I cite this as an indication that he did know the food rules and he did follow what is considered to be a very sensible diet. Of course, eating half a pound to a pound of cheese at a sitting is to me unforgiveable but I'm relating facts. When this happened practically everybody who knew him immediately said, "Oh that was caused by the cheese" and I'm citing this instance to you to lay emphasis on his use of cheese.

In the June 12th, 1970 issue of Science magazine appeared the following abstract.

"Cataracts Produced In Rats By Yogurt — Rats kept on an exclusive diet of yogurt avidly ate the yogurt, grew at a normal rate, were normally active, mated, conceived, and gave birth to normal, healthy litters. However, all of the rats developed cataracts. Cataracts appeared in young rats 2 to 3 months, and in adult rats 4 to 6 months, after initiation of the yogurt diet. Cataracts first manifested themselves in small vacuoles at the periphery of the lens and then in small striae extending toward the center of the lens. These striae progressively became longer, more coarse, and numerous until they coalesced, finally forming a mature white lens. The high content of galactose in commercially available yogurt could account in full for appearance of cataracts in 100 percent of the experimental animals. The cataracts appear to be the same as those produced by diets with a high content of galactose."

"As evidence that cataracts produced by the yogurt

diet result from its high content of galactose is the fact that cataracts produced by yogurt and galactose are clinically indistinguishable."

I must break in here to point out that there is a difference between natural yogurt — or yogurt made in the home or on the farm or the kind of yogurt they used to use back in the olden days or as used throughout the world — and the commercial yogurt sold throughout the food markets in America.

"Yogurt is made from whole milk. The carbohydrate of milk is lactose which breaks down into equal parts of glucose and galactose. Attention is immediately centered on galactose, in view of the findings that a diet with galactose caloric percentage of 22 percent was sufficient to produce cataracts in rats (1). However, in caloric content, galactose comprises only 14.4 percent of whole milk and only 14.2 percent of yogurt made from whole milk (2). Both of these values are well below the cataractogenic level.

"Analysis of the commerically produced yogurt used in our study revealed a much higher content of galactose — from 22 to 24 percent, a value definitely within the cataractogenic range. This striking difference between the galactose content of the commercial yogurt we were using and that of the standard analysis of yogurt prompted us to discuss this discrepancy with the manufacturers of the yogurt.

"We learned that yogurt made in this country is no longer simply the product of fermentative action of the Lactobacillus bulgaricus and Streptococcus thermophilus upon whole milk. Most of the butterfat in the milk is removed before its conversion to yogurt. Removal of butterfat produces a milk which has, relatively speaking, more carbohydrate — and thus more galactose. However, yogurt made from such milk is thin and watery. To

69

improve the consistency, manufacturers add skim milk powder, thus further increasing the caloric percentage of galactose. These procedures account for the elevation of the caloric percentage of galactose in the commercially produced yogurt to cataractogenic level for rats."

Since the appearance of this very important scientific finding there has emerged quite a battle between various factions. Some defend milk and milk products and claim this experiment isn't a fair one because of the fact that the entire diet consisted of yogurt and that this was the only specific instance where yogurt was blamed and that there was no other evidence to support this. However, I refer to the reference in the Yearbook of Agriculture 1959 and I quote accordingly.

"Congenital galactosemia also called galactose diabetes is a disorder in man in which the ability to utilize galactose is low. Infants having this defect show it only after they have been given milk for a few days. The galactose level of the blood rises and the liver becomes enlarged and jaundice occurs. These infants develop cataracts and mental deficiency and may die if they continue to receive only milk.

"The disorder results from the lack of (or lowered activity of) an enzyme necessary for the conversion of galactose to glucose. Infants suffering from this disorder recover quickly if they are given a diet that contains no galactose or lactose.

"Some toxic effects have been observed in animals eating large amounts of lactose, galactose and xylose. The quantities that produce these effects are beyond what a person would normally consume, but because the effects can be produced in animals they deserve consideration.

"Rats fed a diet containing 70 percent of lactose

develop cataracts (the lens of the eye becomes opaque). Galactose and xylose, fed as a large percentage of the diet, also cause cataracts. Galactose and xylose are absorbed but are not readily utilized by the tissues and accumulate in them when they are fed in large quantities. These sugars apparently interfere in some way with the normal utilization of galactose."

In this experiment you will note that the diet of the rats contained only 70% of lactose and they developed cataracts. I would like to remind you of the fact that the experiment was mentioned in the Yearbook of Agriculture for 1959. The book takes more than a year in preparation and the quoted experiment was no doubt done a year or more previous. Thus for over 15 years there has been clear, scientific evidence that dairy products in the human diet do contribute to or cause cataracts.

It is a scientific fact that galactose does not occur naturally in foods. However when milk sugar or lactose is digested, it is broken up into galactose and glucose in the digestive tract.

Galactose is manufactured from milk sugar. However, human tolerance for this sugar (galactose) is limited by the ability of the liver to turn it into glucose. Experiments on rats to judge the ability of the liver or the body to tolerate galactose reveal that the rat apparently has a low tolerance for galactose, and when this type of sugar is fed to rats the galactose content of the blood rises and the eyes develop cataracts.

Experiments indicate that mineral and vitamin deficiencies do not appear to influence the metabolism of galactose and massive doses of vitamins do not change it. It was discovered that a deficiency of protein aggravates the injury caused by galactose, and when high rations of protein were given it showed a definite protective effect.

Therefore, it is clear that galactose should never be used as food and as commercial yogurt contains very high amounts of galactose I point out that it can do nothing but serious harm, especially to the eyes where it positively causes cataracts *(3)*.

I have been studying very carefully some recent experiments conducted by Japanese researchers *(4)*. From these experiments it is clear that whey contains two fractions affecting lactose metabolism: one fraction which prevents cataracts caused by a high lactose diet, but does not markedly improve survival rate or weight gain, and another fraction which improves survival, and increases weight gain, but does not prevent cataracts. Whey, when given to mice eating either the 70 percent lactose or galactose diets, increased survival, but not weight gain. In rats fed the 70 percent galactose diet, whey increased survival and weight gain as well.

Here I want to stress that in this series of experiments the findings are not at all clear but the absence of the whey seems to be very, very important in diet and you must remember that many, if not most, of the commercial dairy products have had the whey eliminated. To the best of my knowledge most cheese, if not all cheese, contains no whey. In the manufacture of yogurt the whole milk is brought to a boil and I would assume that the minerals in the whey have been rendered unassimilable. In any event, I am suggesting that because whey is either absent or impaired in the commercial dairy products this could be an important factor in the causation of cataract.

I would like to quote some figures here that have an interesting sidelight. In 1925 the incidence of short-sightedness or nearsightedness among children in the United States was 25%. In 1935, 10 years later, the incidence jumped to 72%. It is claimed scientifically that this abnormality is associated with a deficiency of calcium or faulty absorption of calcium.

It is claimed that this faulty absorption of calcium allows tension and sometimes spasms of the tiny muscles holding the lens. It is my belief and conviction that this high incidence of short-sightedness and near-sightedness in children is due to the faulty absorption of calcium but the cause in my opinion is clearly established as being due to the pasteurization of milk. Now the big jump from 1925 to 1935 was, I feel, again due to the fact that more milk or most of the milk used during the period was pasteurized. I further maintain that the calcium is rendered unassimilable by the body due to the pasteurization or the use of heat which implies the destruction of the enzymes in the milk.

There are two very interesting papers written by a group of medical researchers. The first one is Galactokinase Deficiency And Cataracts by Norman S. Levy, M.D., Alex E. Krill, M.D., and Ernest Beutler, M.D. The other paper is Cataracts, Galactosuria And Hypergalactosemia Due To Galactokinase Deficiency In A Child by James A. Monteleone, M.D., Ernest Beutler, M.D., Patricia L. Monteleone, M.D., Carmeline L. Utz, B.S., Eliot C. Casey, M.D.

There appears to be ample proof to clearly indicate that galactose is not only suspect but actually guilty. Galactose according to the dictionary is a mono sacharide or simple hexose sugar. Galactose is an isomer of glucose and it is formed along with glucose in the hydrolisis of lactose. Galactose is what is known as milk sugar and it is a di-sacharide which on hydrolisis yields glucose and galactose. I suspect that the changes effected in milk and milk products due to pasteurization may be a factor in creating the problem.

Galactokinase is the enzyme that breaks down the galactose and which makes it assimilable by the body. In the formation of galactose or lactose, enzymes are involved. From my studies of enzymes I learned that enzymes are readily destroyed by heat. Therefore, in the pasteurization process or in other manufacturing processes the galactose enzyme (galactokinase) would suffer or be completely destroyed, thus creating the galactokinase deficiency which appears to be the main cause of congenital and probably other forms of cataract. I want it clearly understood that I'm not trying to build a case against dairy products. All I'm seeking is the truth and I will go to any length to obtain it.

DAIRY PRODUCTS AND THE
FINDINGS FROM 'CITY OF HOPE'

A geneticist at the City of Hope Hospital in Los Angeles, Calif., tells us that children and young adults who have cataracts caused by an inherited metabolic defect can be helped by putting them on a milk free diet. Dr. Ernest Beutler, chairman of the Division of Medicine at the City of Hope tells us that the particular genetic defect at fault is a deficiency of the enzymes used by the body to metabolize galactose sugar. Then he tells us "This kind of sugar is found in many foods but milk, ice cream, yogurt and other milk products are especially high in it". He goes on to further tell us that if the enzyme galactokinase is absent from the body, or present in insufficient quantities, galactose sugar cannot be used properly, and the lens of the eye is affected.

Then he makes this important statement — "When milk products are removed from the diet the cataracts are kept from getting worse and, in some cases actually improved." This project is sponsored by the National Genetic Foundation as well as other agencies for the aid of the blind. The galactokinase assay is a complicated biochemical procedure being done only at a few medical centres. We learn from this research that about 15 million

74

Americans are afflicted with genetic disorders of one kind or another. Dr. Beutler is Director of the National Genetics Foundation's Counselling and Treatment Centre at the City of Hope *(5)*.

REFERENCES

1. Mitchell, H.S., and Hodges, W.M., ibid. 9, 37 (1935).

2. Bridges, M.A., Food And Beverage Analysis (Lea and Febiger, Philadelphia, 1935).

3. Food And Life, Yearbook of Agriculture, 1939, pg. 153.

4. Tamura, S., Tsuzuki, S., and Masuda, M., Journal of Pharmacology 21: 107, 1971.

5. Los Angeles Times, Monday, Sept. 4, 1972.

6 Cataract and Old Age

From my broad reading of medical literature it is clear that organized medicine takes the view that degenerative or senile cataract, which is by far the most common type of cataract, is a disease or condition of old age. The origin of this idea or belief is not too hard to find because it so happens that many older people, in fact a fairly high percentage of old people, do have cataracts or have had them removed.

It is my belief that the medical profession state that cataract is a disease of old age simply because they claim there is neither any cause nor any cure of this most alarming disease. So attributing it to old age is about the easiest and the most natural way to get out from under. So when someone with cataracts asks why and how the doctor just shrugs his shoulders and says, "Old age". And that could apply to anyone who is more than 50 years of age. It so happens that I know a great number of people in their 60's, 70's, 80's and even in their 90's who live within the ideas and scope that I recommend and none of them has cataracts or glaucoma. Furthermore, from my studies of the centenarians (those people over 100 years of age) very few of them were afflicted with cataract.

It goes without saying that older people have more cataracts than younger people percentage-wise and, by the same token, they have practically every other disease in greater percentage than young people and that's using only plain, simple mathematics. For example, Dr. Ochsner, the famed surgeon who specializes in lung cancer operations, says with a ring of authority that every person who smokes will eventually get cancer of the lungs if he lives long enough. No one can deny the truth of that statement but in his case he specifies clearly that you have to be a smoker. By the same token, if you live to be 100 years of age in the conventional manner the chances are very high that you will have a cataract.

It is my serious belief that cataract will affect those of old age if they live in such a way so that cataract will result. That is, their dietary and living habits and other conditions make for cataracts. Like most other degenerative diseases, and senile cataract is definitely a degenerative disease, cataract takes time to happen and the older we get the greater are the chances of cataract. But, by the same token, those of us who live so as to prevent cataract would be no more likely to get cataract at 80 than at 20 or 50. So if you live right and eat right and do things that will prevent cataracts, whether you're 18 or 80, I don't think you'll ever become afflicted with them.

I have made rather exhaustive studies to see if there was any positive link between cataract and old age and I want to assure you with all the rhetoric at my command that there is no link whatsoever. Please believe me, I am a reporter and if there was a link I would say so. I have no desire or wish to hide any information. There are, no doubt, many degenerative conditions and deformities and illnesses that do tend to afflict older people but cataract is definitely not one of them. So just because you are living to be older is no reason that you will be afflicted with cataracts. Again I ask you to accept this as a positive, empirical and scientific statement.

However, my studies have revealed that there are positive, specific, causative factors of cataract. But it depends upon the frequency of these habits and the extent of the biological, mechanical and drug violations as to how soon the cataract will result.

Enzymes are essential for general health. It is a known scientific fact that as we grow older our bodies have fewer and fewer enzymes. We know that the enzyme count drops as we get older, we know that cataract effects people as they get older. Enzymes are found only in living food. I'm suggesting there is a connection. Make sure that you get foods, whole foods, live foods containing enzymes and then the chances of developing cataract are lessened if not entirely eliminated. So you can still be old and have your full quota of enzymes by eating adequate quantities of raw vegetables, raw grains and raw fruit.

Various clear patterns became evident in my studies and if you adopt and follow the cataract-creating pattern, and stick with it closely, you will be sure to be afflicted with cataracts.

I go on record as stating with absolute certainty that your chance of developing cataracts depends entirely on what you do or what you do not do to create them Cataract never attacked anyone out of a clear blue sky. There must have been contributing causes or factors. Furthermore, cataract is not something that is wished upon or inflicted upon anyone by nature or an unseen power or a nasty human-hating devil or deity. There is no doubt that cataract is earned, cataract is created by contributing factors and malfunction of the animal organism.

Now here is a very important statement and I beg that you take note of it. I wish to assure all people, but especially those who are passing middle age and into the retirement bracket that cataract is not inevitable and, what's more important, if you do not have cataracts at the present time then you can be sure never to have them if you follow the sane proper living habits, especially the dietary habits, suggested and recommended in this book.

I know and mention other important considerations in cataract . . . but this is by far the most vital factor of all.

I don't know how to make it any stronger, I don't know how to word it any more clearly but I want it emblazoned far and wide to all who wish to prevent cataracts that all they need do to avoid ever having them is to follow my nutritional advice and avoid the cataract-causing traits and habits.

7 Diabetes and Cataract

There appears to be a definite link between diabetes and cataract and a lesser link with glaucoma. Just how strong the link is has not as yet been established but it appears that both diabetes and cataract result from similar dietary habits. Now researchers can pinpoint at least one of the more important diabetic causes as poor, refined or concentrated carbohydrates. There is research evidence that seems to indicate that cataract sufferers have a low carbohydrate intake. It is generally assumed that diabetic people have a high carbohydrate intake but my investigations reveal that these are invariably refined carbohydrates. Whole carbohydrate foods are seldom used anywhere in America.

Medical science tells us that high blood sugar is the mark of a diabetic. It is believed that diabetics have an excess of ketone acids in their blood and it appears that these acids cause the graying of the lens. In experiments when the lens has been incubated with ketone acids the lens becomes gray and this graying of the lens is what we know as cataract. An eminent authority on diabetes informed me that "Cataracts can be caused by excess ketones which the diabetic makes when he has no insulin. Or the normal makes on a low carbohydrate diet". They also found that an excess of galactose in the blood will produce the same result . . . that is, graying of the lens. Professor Groen of Israel has incubated the eye lens of animals in ketones and has found that cataracts were formed. This would clearly indicate that ketones are positively involved in the formation of cataracts.

I wish to explain that ketone acids in the body are the end products of metabolism. The presence of ketosis is easily determined by testing for the presence of acitone or diacetic acid in the urine. First ketosis appears in the blood and when this reaches an elevated level, evidence of acidosis in diabetes reaches measurable proportions in the urine. Thus ketonuria is one of the early bits of evidence indicating acidosis in diabetes.

As mentioned earlier rats do develop cataracts when on a commercial yogurt diet. Studies have revealed that commercial yogurt contains almost double the amount of galactose of the natural or homemade yogurt, 24% against 14%. It is established that this increase is due to the various chemicals added in the process of commercial yogurt manufacture. Obviously the so-called improved method is necessary to increase, speed up the process and make it more pleasing to the taste. Both citric and lactic acids have been used along with other less natural chemicals to speed up the manufacture of this once natural, useful dairy product.

It is also known that a low or refined, processed carbohydrate diet appears to cause an excess of ketones. It is my calculated opinion — and I stress it — that only the refined, processed and concentrated carbohydrates bring about this condition. When you eat only whole carbohydrates these conditions will not appear. I believe we now have the link between commercial, processed dairy products, milk, galactose, diet, cataracts and diabetes.

The following is an article of interest.

"Young rats were made diabetic by injection of alloxan and comparable groups of them were maintained on different types of diets. Three diets had a beneficial effect. The time of appearance of cataracts was significantly delayed by a high choline diet, by a diet without fat, and by a diet containing 0.2% a-tocopherol *(1)*."

It appears that many or most diabetics have eye disorders. All of the diabetics I have known in my life have had trouble of some form or another with their eyes. One estimation by a knowledgeable authority was that more than half of all diabetics have either glaucoma or cataract. I further maintain that even if diabetics do not have any indication of eye disorders in the early days of the disease, there is a strong possibility that the trouble will appear.

So this forces me to ask a rather pointed question. Is there some condition in a diabetic's body, be it ketones, galactose, the insulin itself or even some factor connected with insulin that is antagonistic to or destroys riboflavin? Or if not the riboflavin, some other nutrient that nourishes or supports the eye, or maybe more specifically the lens? It could be the ketones.

Granted there are people who have glaucoma or cataracts and are not diabetics. Still I feel it would be worth studying and ascertaining whether these people who have cataracts and glaucoma or other disorders are borderline diabetics or are leaning towards that condition.

There appears to be little if any doubt that cataracts and glaucoma are nutritional or deficiency diseases. I'm suspecting that an over-supply of something can create a deficiency in the same way as the process of osmosis wherein the stronger solution depletes the weaker. This is established in horticulture, where if your soil is too rich it will draw out the few nutrients that are in the plant or plant roots and deplete the plant and cause it injury or death. I am suggesting that there could be such a relationship in diabetes, cataract and glaucoma.

REFERENCES

1. Charalampous, F.C., and Hegsted, D.M. Effect of age and diet on development of cataracts in the diabetic rat. Am. J. Physiol. 161, 540-4, 1950.

8 The Eyes and Headache

I recall in my youth, probably from the age of 10 upwards, whenever any child had a headache almost invariably the child wound up being fitted with glasses. Even when I was ten years of age I had headaches but, partly because my parents didn't have money and partly because I didn't complain, I never got glasses. I know I'm a nasty man but I would be willing to wager my life that 75% of all young people or children who were fitted with glasses because of headaches never needed the glasses, but do need them today because their eyes have been weakened so that glasses are absolutely necessary if they are to see.

I have been fighting this battle of headaches and the eyes and glasses for well over 50 years but it hasn't got me anywhere. More and more people wear glasses, more and more children and young people are fitted with glasses . . . so I'm not doing very well in my crusade. Just how many conditions there are that cause headaches I do not know but it has been estimated that there are well over 25 different conditions, diseases or illnesses that cause headaches.

I am suggesting that irrespective of the actual cause of the headache, when you are young the diagnosis will usually be that you need glasses and you will eventually wear them.

I am fully aware that I will be disliked, hated, ridiculed and cursed by thousands of oculists, optometrists, ophthalmologists and physicians in general and especially by the people who make the lens and the frame but observations for almost 50 years cannot be kicked over or cast aside easily. I will stick to my guns and repeat that most young people are forced to wear glasses unnecessarily.

Granted, poor nutrition which is widespread throughout America, does tend to weaken the eyes and lessen vision but still the answer is not glasses. I further claim that most of the headaches that are treated and diagnosed as eye trouble are not necessarily that but it is an easy way out and one that is very acceptable. The best proof on earth that I can offer of the validity of my assertion is that most people who wear glasses still take aspirin and many other pain relieving drugs to stop or relieve their headaches. What I'm saying is simply that wearing glasses does not remove the headache. When you wear glasses and you have headaches you go to your doctor and, seeing you are wearing glasses, the doctor can no longer prescribe glasses . . . he instead prescribes aspirin or some other analgesic drug.

I will not deny that at times eye strain or other visional problems may cause a headache or contribute to one but just because strain or some other defect of the eyes causes a headache does not necessarily mean that glasses are the answer. Remember, usually when you put glasses on a child it is forever because the eyes from that moment onward are weakened and as he grows older the eyes become weaker and the glasses become thicker. Investigate, look around and see whether or not I speak the truth. Obviously I am casting reflections upon the honesty and the integrity and ethics concerning the various practitioners because I'm involving medical doctors, opticians and ophthalmologists. But I claim that glasses and eye examinations and eye treatments are their stock in trade and I am rat enough to suggest that 'business is business'. After all, a large percentage of the people of America wear glasses, so what . . . so another one wears glasses! People who wear glasses are a good source of income to these various professions and trades. A person who does not wear glasses does not contribute to their welfare.

One of the strongest arguments against the use of glasses is the fact that by their magnification they lessen the work or the effort of the eye muscles. It is my positive contention that organs become strong and flexible by doing the work for which they were originally intended not by having their work done for them by various or devious means. I further maintain that this holds emphatically true for the eyes and their muscles. Therefore, glasses or eye crutches should only be used as a last resort when nutritional means and eye exercise have failed to produce the desired results. I will further state that this will rarely happen. It is also important that you remember that these eye exercises must be continued all the days of your life. In my opinion glasses pervert the natural functions of the eye muscles and cause them to lose their mobility and to atrophy. Glasses force nature to depend upon mechanical props which is not good.

The simple truth is that glasses are unnatural. They are crutches, they are clear-cut proof that the physician or the healer is incapable of correcting your condition. Therefore, he gives you a pair of crutches to hobble along with for the rest of your life. I am regarded as a scourge by most healers and I'm telling you this . . . if you go to visit a urologist you will in about 90% of the cases wind up with surgery. If you go to a healer or a medical doctor in general you will wind up with a prescription and drugs and if you consult an eye doctor or an eye man be he an optometrist, optician or ophthalmologist the chances are about 95 to 5 that you'll wind up wearing glasses.

Here are a few interesting sidelights about the optical trade and profession which were brought to light recently by reporters investigating the eye glass business.

"In Los Angeles, a wily reporter made his own investigation. Barry Siegle, of L.A. Newspaper, went to five different optometrists and received five different prescriptions for glasses. Three of the prescriptions varied an entire measuring level weaker or stronger, and the other two were even further apart."

Another reporter learned that "An optometrist goes through four years of training, a true eye doctor, an ophthalmologist, has 13 years of schooling, including an M.D. degree. The difference between an optometrist and an ophthalmologist is the difference between a midwife and an obstetrician."

A reporter for Consumer Newsletter found that "Some examiners faked tests by flashing lights in the patient's eyes. In the Jersey study, 88% of the customers received the wrong glasses, including those with perfect vision who were fitted with window glass."

The reporters discovered that the medical doctors or ophthalmologists never referred patients to optometrists. Now in fairness to the optometrical profession I would like to state that this was not necessarily due to the fact that they did not regard optometrists as being capable craftsman. First let me state they regard optometrists as competition and perhaps the optometrists did not kick back large percentages of their sales to the ophthalmologist like the optometrical house or the optician does. There is no use denying or being surprised at the fact that the ophthalmologists receive these kickbacks because it has been positively and clearly established that the ophthalmologists do get these kickbacks, or did get them, and they amounted to vast sums of money so let's be fair to the optometrists. Maybe they don't get the ophthalmologists' business because they don't give the eye doctors a rake-off.

You may defend the various eye specialists by stating they are eye doctors and not nutritionists or counsellors and thus it is not their duty or function to direct your diet or way of life. However, I am of the old fashioned school and feel that we are our brother's keeper and therefore they should tell young people especially, to correct their diet instead of prescribing glasses which destroy or weaken their eyes permanently.

Lately the news media, especially the newspapers and magazines, have been filled with articles commending and flattering the medical profession for their tremendous advances in the past year. I have checked carefully through the list and I would suggest that they are not advances . . . they are backward steps. In spite of all the so-called advances even qualified medical men admit that very little if anything has been accomplished regarding vision, eyes, cataract, glaucoma and other eye diseases. They claim to have improved the surgical techniques in cataract. Just how well this will work out will not be known for some years because it takes many hundreds or many thousands of guinea pigs to prove or disprove something when it pertains to health in human beings. But as for any worthwhile research findings concerning the health and the well being of the eyes and vision, absolutely nothing has come to light. Therefore, anyone with trouble with his eyes had better not hold his breath waiting for some new medical advance to alleviate or correct his condition.

Here we find a very interesting article concerning eyestrain and headache and it was taken from a book entitled "Principles Of Internal Medicine".

"Eyestrain. Errors of refraction of the eyes are a well-recognized cause of headache. In such cases pain tends to be referred to the orbit, forehead, and temple, does not throb with the pulse, and tends to occur during intensive use of the eyes as in reading or close work, and to persist for some time afterward. It is particularly obtrusive toward evening, and if the subject is fatigued. There is evidence to show that in the presence of refractive error, use of the eyes produces sustained contraction of the extraocular muscles of the orbit, and of the frontal, temporal, and even occipital muscles, and it is suggested that the pain results from this contraction. A similar mechanism is postulated for the headache of glaucoma. The relief of such refractive errors by use of the correct spectacles abolishes the headache. *Headache from eyestrain is probably not as frequent as would be indicated by the number of spectacles prescribed for its relief. (Italics Ours)* Hyperopic astigmatism is a more frequent cause than myopia *(1)*."

As one so-called eye expert phrases it, "Perhaps no condition more frequently leads to the conclusion of eyestrain than headache."

He goes on to say that most people immediately blame their headache on their eyes. This is often justifiable since refractive errors and muscular defects will produce headache symptoms. In these instances he goes on to tell us the pain is spoken of as dull or drawing along the brow and in or between the eyes. These headaches are aggravated by movies, television, reading or sewing. He suggests that headaches resulting from car-sickness or train-sickness are to some degree due to eyestrain. He suggests that muscular defects and astigmatism predispose to headache. He also claims glare and annoying reflections produce headaches as well as glaucoma in which case a dull ache may become excruciating. He suggests that frontal headaches are commonly caused by eyestrain and that temporal headaches and those at the back of the head and neck are frequently caused by eyestrain and generally by astigmatism, muscular defect and excessive glare.

Glaucoma, iritis and iridis cause frontal pain and pain at the back of the eye. Among the other causes he mentions giddiness, sinus conditions and allergies, diabetes as well as low blood sugar.

I've come across information that "the deficiency in vitamin A can cause headaches, photophobia (fear and sensitivity to light), burning and itching of the eyes."

Dr. Harold M. Peppard, author of "Sight Without Glasses", claims that the eyes are seldom the primary cause of headaches. He also suggests that "unfailing relief is realized when the patient is instructed in the principles of normal sight. If the headache is not relieved by this treatment one can be absolutely certain that it is not the eyes but some other part of the head or body that is causing the headache".

Dr. Peppard cites a case — "A few months ago a young woman came to me with a history of severe headaches for the past two years. During that time she had had several eye examinations and she wore glasses, but with only slight relief from her headaches. On examining her eyes carefully, I could not see anything there that should cause headaches.

"It was a delicate situation, since the patient had been sent to me by another physician who expected me to confine myself to the eyes. Nevertheless, I questioned her on her general health, diet, elimination, amount of sleep, type and extent of activity, because I knew that this woman did not need to wear glasses and that the cause of her headache was not in her eyes. The trouble was uncovered. A simple but complete change of diet cured her headaches and also enabled her to take off her glasses and leave them off."

He goes on — "Unfortunately, in some cases, the glasses relieve the headache sufficiently to lead the patient to believe that it is the eyes that are the real cause of the trouble.

"To illustrate further the necessity of a careful diagnosis in headache, the following case may serve to bring out an additional point of some importance: A young man came for an eye examination with these symptoms: headache, eyeache, stomach trouble in the form of excessive gas. He had been examined by two good eye specialists and was at the time under the care of a stomach specialist.

"I removed his glasses, which had been worn for two years, and gave him the eye treatment. In a few weeks his vision had returned to normal and his eyes on examination showed no evidence of the former astigmatism. But the pain in the eyes and the headaches, though a bit better, were still present.

"Anyone doing this kind of eye work can be positive in his diagnosis as to whether or not the trouble is in the eyes. In spite of the pain there, I knew that the cause was not there. That settled, we were able to explore along a different path. Again it was the diet. That was radically changed and all of his remaining symptoms were cleared up.

"These cases drive home the fact that headache is a difficult condition to diagnose. To assume that the eyes cause the trouble is a great error, far too common among the specialists in their respective lines.

"The thing that misleads one is that the eyes feel sensitive or weak or hurt when they are used and so they are blamed for the trouble, while all the time it is the cause of the headache that makes the eyes sensitive.

"When the oculist puts glasses on one of these cases, he is not doing any more to relieve the cause of the headache than a man does when he takes an aspirin. In each case the symptom, not the cause, is being treated, and the alleviation of the symptom makes it just that much more difficult to locate the cause of the trouble.

"If this knowledge were more generally known and recognized it would put a stop to this vicious habit of putting glasses on children and adults because they have headaches."

I have learned, through my observations and study, one of the principal causes of headaches. Believe it or not, they can be caused or brought about by the eyes but can be readily corrected without the use of glasses. It is my belief that the keenest students, the most mentally alert young people and children suffer from headaches due to eyestrain. At least that is what is given as the cause but it is not eyestrain. These intense, alert, bright young people become tense and tend to strain because of their keen interest in what their teacher or lecturer is telling them and they focus their eyes upon the teacher and hardly remove them for many minutes at a time. I suggest that this causes eyestrain because the eyes are not moving about, which they should do, and therefore headaches are the result. So it has nothing to do with the eyes and to prescribe glasses for situations like this is a tragedy and does serious harm. It would be better and more sensible to teach the child or the individual to relax his eyes. He can still have his mind and his ears alerted but teach the child to shift his eyes so

93

that eyestrain will not be the result — and then no headaches.

It is strange that seldom is this very important fact made clear to parents and I strongly advocate proper instructions so as to negate the need for glasses because of this particular kind of headache caused by intensive staring and strain.

It was Dr. William Horatio Bates who taught that whenever you are looking at anything be it a view, a date calendar, the page of a book or a person it should have the effect of allowing the vision to come to you in a more or less relaxed fashion or a relaxed eye and never should the eye be allowed to become tense and reach out after anything. It is this concentrated strain or staring that causes a headache and this must be corrected. So do not permit yourself to strain or stare, and learn to blink or close the eyes for a few seconds regularly. This will prevent you from staring and thus causing headaches.

Obviously the manufacture and the sale of glasses is big business involving millions upon millions of dollars annually in America. The use and the prescribing of glasses is serious enough but putting on a campaign to sell sunglasses — which are with rare exceptions unnecessary but which we are taught and made to believe that we need — is, in my opinion, a crime. I would like to quote from some of the literature distributed by the optical companies, the opticians or the optometrists in order to do more business or make a sale.

"Cataract is not an unusual occurrence after age 50, and after 65 is the foremost cause of blindness. Any opacity of the human lens is cataract. Milky white scar tissue on the front surface of the eye is not cataract. Some cataracts grow rapidly, other slowly. Some remain stationary, others are absorbed. Some exist at birth, others come only with advanced age.

"Cataract may be caused by injury, radium, X-rays, atomic radiation, Electric shock, lightning, explosion, systemic disorders, old age and infrared radiation. Except for old age, infrared light is the most frequent cause of cataract. Fortunately infrared radiation is the one thing that can be controlled insofar as it influences the development of cataract.

"Infrared rays cause cataract because heat or infrared radiation coagulates protein, the human lens contains a higher percentage of protein than any other organ of the body, coagulated protein is opaque, and opaque protein in the human lens is cataract. Thus the change which takes place in the protein of the human lens when it is exposed to the heat of infrared radiation is similar to the change which takes place in the white of an egg exposed to the heat of cooking.

"It is common knowledge that cataract develops early, rapidly and with high frequency in countries where light and heat are intense. It is equally well known that glassblowers, metal workers, stokers, and others similarly exposed to intense light and heat risk developing cataract prematurely. Although relatively few of us are exposed to such extreme climatic and occupational risks, many of us do expose our eyes to the harmful infrared radiation that lurks in the light reflected from bright skies and white clouds, hot sandy beaches, glittering water, tennis courts and glary roadways. Most of us know that exposure of our eyes to such extremely bright light is unpleasant and harmful and accordingly use some kind of sunglasses to offset the danger.

"But, 'there's the rub' — what kind of sunglasses?"

I beg to differ with the big build up for sunglasses

warning you of the grave dangers in the sun, "Many of us do expose our eyes to the harmful infrared radiation that lurks in the light reflected from bright skies and white clouds, hot sandy beaches, glittering water, tennis courts and glary roadways." Personally I am convinced that the sun brings great benefits to the eye and can only do harm if recklessly abused. Furthermore, the vitamin D so essential for eye health would be eliminated or reduced if sunglasses were worn. Therefore sunglasses actually do much more harm than good. So here we have it. The eye doctors and lens sellers are going all out to sell you still another harmful pair of glasses . . . one isn't enough. They would like to have you visit them like you visit your doctor, the more often the better for their business.

Here we have a real high pressure pitch from their bag of literature.

"This brings us to that one thing worth knowing about cataract, namely: The potentially harmful infrared radiation of ordinary sunlight may be eliminated by properly prescribed absorptive lenses. Conversely, and of high import, this is not true of the cheap substandard sunglasses so thoughtlessly purchased by an unsuspecting public. Such sunglasses, aside from lacking discriminative absorptive qualities, contain other imperfections which strain all eyes and seriously harm some. Proper protective absorptive lenses are of particular importance to those whose occupation, hobby or recreational activities involve exposure to bright sunlight where there is always some danger of infrared radiation predisposing the eyes to premature cataract.

"When we go fishing, hunting, swimming, iceskating, sailing, motoring, golfing, or skiing most of us go elaborately and expensively equipped with the paraphernalia of the sport involved, BUT all too many of us completely overlook that relatively inexpensive item — properly prescribed sunglasses to protect our eyes from the infrared radiation inherent in the light under which all such activities are carried on.

"All of which means that everyone, no matter what his calling or avocations, should be provided with properly prescribed sunglasses to protect the eyes against the potentially harmful, cataract-causing infrared radiation present in all sunlight everywhere. This advice, if heeded, especially by those who are likely to reach a ripe old age, may help insure clear, comfortable, efficient and happy seeing to the very end."

My findings are that sunglasses of any kind do not protect a healthy eye. Sunglasses always prevent normal visual acuity and prevent essential, beneficial rays from reaching the eye.

It should be a criminal offence to sell sunglasses.

REFERENCES

1. Principles of Internal Medicine, 2nd Edition, 1954, pg. 23.

9 Cataract Surgery

To begin with I will quote several medical opinions concerning cataract surgery.

"Surgery is the only known effective treatment for cataract. Patients should not be misled by the claims of quacks or charlatans that 'magic' salves, drops or pills will dissolve a cataract; it cannot now be done. Cataract surgery, while a delicate and serious operation, is safe and successful more than 95 times out of 100 among those persons for whom surgery is recommended. Cataract patients may approach surgical treatment with every confidence and anticipation of regaining useful vision."

"The only known cure for cataract is surgical removal. No pill, eye drop, injection, or any other substance or procedure will correct or prevent cataracts."

"There are no known drops or medicines that will dissolve cataracts. However, much of the incidence of blindness due to a cataract can be prevented through early detection, eventual removal of the cataract through surgery, and the post-surgical use of prescription lenses. Prescribing and use of contact lenses by optometrists in correcting vision following cataract removal has contributed to the full rehabilitation of many affected cataract patients, enabling them to return to work, hobbies and normal living."

"A person operated on for cataracts must wear corrective lenses for the rest of his life. A pair of special glasses or contact lenses is necessary to replace the clouded lens removed from the eye."

"Cataract is a condition in which the crystalline lens clouds over until it becomes opaque, blocking out vision. Cataract can afflict anyone and may be caused by a number of things. Usually, however, it results from the ageing process and most often occurs in people over fifty. The remedy is to remove the lens surgically and to replace its lost power with glasses or contact lenses."

From the latest figures it appears that there will be in the year 1973 approximately 500,000 cataract extractions in America and that there will be close to 10 percent complications following the cataract extraction. This figure appears to be higher than that given earlier by authorities who claim practically 95 percent success.

Speaking generally, cataract surgery removes the crystalline lens, the function of which is to enable the eye to focus on objects at various distances. After surgery one must wear extra special glasses with a built-in lens to take the place of the crystalline lens that was removed in surgery. These must be worn for the rest of one's life. The use of this cataract lens does not restore side vision . . . actually, it means the loss of side vision. I suggest this is somewhat similar to a horse wearing blinkers so he can't see to the side, just straight ahead. As yet medical science has not found any way or means of providing for side vision and one must be content seeing straight ahead

100

and at best being able to read in varying fashion.

Medical science in general terms claims that better than 95% of cataract surgery is successful. Please bear in mind that the surgeon's or the physician's interpretation of successful is at variance with the term successful as generally used outside of the medical profession. I've heard hundreds of times, and you no doubt have heard many times the statement that the operation was a success but the patient died . . . of complications . . . nothing whatsoever to do with the surgery. This is the general pattern established from the results of operations or surgery. But there is no doubt that there are skilled surgeons thoroughly capable in every way and who actually fulfill their promise. If they say they can successfully remove your prostate or cataract they can perform this function and there is no one who can dispute it. However, the results after the surgery sometimes do not fulfill the promise of the surgeon or the expectations of the individual upon whom the operation was performed.

For many years I failed to grasp the significance of the positive statement that better than 95% of cataract surgery was successful. What is clearly meant is that in 95% of the cases the 'lens' is removed without complications. Here is the clincher . . . it does not mean that 95% vision will be restored after surgery. Yet when a surgeon guarantees 95% success in cataract operations the poor patient believes he has a 95% chance of regaining his vision. No one attempts to correct the illusion.

An ophthalmologist on the staff of a Massachusetts Eye and Ear Infirmary and Harvard Medical School states "In certain instances a cataract should be removed even though vision in the better eye is still excellent. The patient must be guided by his physician's advice, and should not let himself become inactive because of poor vision. Neither age nor the state of general health need deter a patient from surgery, since cataract extraction under local anesthesia can be very rewarding visually and without hazard even to a frail patient.

"It is not unusual for a person 90 years old or more to undergo successful cataract extraction, and to be gratified at the wisdom of his decision to do so."

"After the operation one or both eyes will be bandaged and covered with a protective shield. You will stay in bed, quiet and relaxed, for at least twenty-four hours, avoiding any straining motions. Your eyes will remain covered for as long as your surgeon believes necessary for your safety. If, when the anesthetic wears off, you begin to feel a dull ache, you will call the nurse and ask for medicine to prevent this discomfort. Pain can make you restless, and therefore endanger the eye. So, don't try to be a hero — ask the nurse for help if your eye begins to hurt. Ask the nurse to help shift your position in bed if your back becomes tired — don't try to do this yourself.

"While your eyes are covered, you will be fed by someone, first liquids, then soft foods, then a regular diet according to your doctor's orders. At an appropriate time your surgeon will remove the bandages and gently cleanse the eyes, using suitable eyedrops or salve. He will leave uncovered one or both eyes at the proper time, depending on your progress, and soon you will be allowed to sit up, first on the edge of the bed, then in a chair at the bedside. A little later you will be allowed to go to the bathroom and walk in the corridor with an attendant to watch over you at first.

THINGS TO REMEMBER IN THE HOSPITAL

1. Don't put your hands up to your face.

2. Don't move head, arms or legs rapidly. Move slowly and without strain.

3. Don't bend over or stoop down.

4. Don't lift anything.

5. Don't shave or comb your hair until the doctor gives you permission.

6. Don't tie your shoes — wear slippers into which you can slide your feet.

7. Don't strain while moving your bowels.

"Your eyes will run tears and be sensitive to light for a while after cataract removal. Any sticky secretion will be removed by your doctor on his daily visits. He may order dark glasses to lessen discomfort from sensitivity to light. If you expect to see clearly the minute your bandages are removed you will be disappointed. Only when the eye has healed suitably will your doctor allow you to ease gently into the wearing of those special eyeglasses which are necessary to good vision after removal of a cataract. Sometimes the first glasses are called 'temporary' because they are followed weeks or months later by permanent glasses.

"Only your doctor knows when it will be safe for you to leave the hospital. You will arrange for someone to take you home, for it is not safe for you to go by yourself. Someone must carry your suitcase for you, and the driver of the car must be instructed to go slowly and smoothly, avoiding bumps and sudden stops.

"For about two months after your cataract has been removed, your doctor will want you to avoid anything which could press on your eye, or any strain which could damage it. During the convalescent period of three months or so, he is entirely dependent on your co-operation; for the success of your operation now depends on you. Your doctor will probably want you to pay careful attention to the following advice, until he tells you otherwise:

103

1. Let others wait on you — you would do the same for them if they were in your position.

2. Keep your hands away from your face and head as much as possible.

3. Do not hold children or permit them to be near you — or animals either.

4. Do not lift anything weighing more than a pound or two, and then only from a table high enough so you do not have to bend over.

5. Do not stoop to pick up anything for any reason at all; and do not bend to put on or tie your shoes. Wear house slippers that you can slip into easily.

6. Move slowly at all times, and walk only in familiar and well-lighted places where you are less liable to bump something or fall.

7. Do not strain when you go to the toilet. If you are having trouble, ask your physician for a mild laxative that will keep you from straining.

8. Wash your face gently with a damp washcloth, keeping far away from your eyes. Don't bend over the wash basin or slosh water in your face.

9. Do not brush your teeth for the first few weeks but use mouthwash instead. When you do start to brush the teeth, do so gently, without any violent head motions.

10. Do not comb your hair except by special permission of your physician.

11. Put your glasses on very carefully, as the tips of the side pieces may poke you in the eye if

you are careless. Hold the glasses by these tips when putting them on.

12. Wear dark glasses when you are in bright sunlight or in a place where the light is very bright, if they make you more comfortable. A broad-brimmed hat will help you when you are outside, and pulling the shades will help inside.

"Mild discomfort, tearing, aches or pains are not unusual. If pain is relieved by two aspirin tablets (Empirin, or Bufferin, etc.), it is probably not important pain. But persistent aching, or change in vision, or any marked change in how you feel should be reported at once to your doctor (or, if he is not immediately available, to his nurse or secretary) so that you may be examined without delay.

"Do not attempt to clean your operated eye yourself, but have someone else do it for you: Have this person boil water vigorously for ten minutes, and then allow it to cool to room temperature for an hour. Then the attendant should wash his hands, wet a piece of sterile cotton with the cooled water, and gently wipe only the edges of the lids, and only enough to remove the sticky mucus. In doing this, the attendant's finger should rest upon the cheekbone as he gently parts the lids by pulling down the lower lid. If drops are ordered, follow the same procedure as in washing. Have the attendant gently pull down the lower lid, resting his finger on your cheekbone while you lean back slightly and look at the ceiling. The attendant should bring the dropper towards the eye from the side away from the nose, and allow one drop to run into the corner of the eye. No harm will be done by using more than one drop.

"After the eyes have healed, normal sight — or close to it — can be expected in most cases unless some other eye disease in addition to cataract has been present. After a normal convalescence, usually about 3 months in duration,

105

you can expect your physician to find your eyes fit for you to return to your work, whether you are a proof reader, secretary, taxi driver, switchboard operator or whatever, with the possible exception of work entailing heavy manual labor, or precarious footing.

"Removal of the lens from your eye means that the eye itself no longer has the ability to bend light rays to form an image. Eyeglasses must be worn to bring you clear vision. These 'cataract glasses' must be very carefully adjusted by the fitter, for they must be worn at exactly the proper distance from the eye if you are to see clearly. It will take a short time to become accustomed to your new glasses. Objects will appear larger than before, and you will find yourself reaching for things only to find them a little beyond your grasp. Door frames and other long straight lines may seem curved.

"Optical advances have occurred in recent years along with surgical advances. Spectacle lenses for cataract patients no longer need be so weighty as formerly. The newer type glasses are more accurate in their image formation, and are designed to make available a wider expanse of side vision than did earlier lens formulas."

I'd like to quote from a book called "You and Your Eyes" by Lawrence Lewison.

"Modern-day cataract surgery is responsible for the restoration of useful sight to many eyes, and has become an operative procedure almost as routine as tonsillectomy and appendectomy. Lens extraction causes the eye to become very far-sighted, because approximately 13 Diopters of power are eliminated. A strong convex lens must then be applied in order to bring images into proper focus."

The two principle types of lens extraction are intracapsular and extracapsular. The former is where the lens is removed totally . . . I mean with the lens still contained in its original capsule. However, in the extracapsular surgery the front portion of the capsule is first ruptured and removed. Then the lens cortex and nucleus are taken from the eye, leaving the rear portion of the capsule where it was. The reason that this procedure is used is that it is easier to perform than the intracapsular lens extraction method. However, in time a secondary membrane forms which has to be removed later in about one-third of the cases.

Let us assume that you are resigned to the fact, or convinced by your doctor, that you should undergo cataract surgery. Let me make a suggestion and it may well be worth your while to listen to this suggestion. Go out and find at least five people who have had cataract extraction. Now don't go to ones that the surgeon sends you to but dig up these individuals by yourself through inquiry, through friends and other sources. It is your duty to find at least five people who have had this surgery and then ask them straight-forward to give you their opinion and their advice. Then and then only make your decision as to whether or not you will have the cataract surgery.

Now let us look at the latest surgical techniques.

There is a new type of surgery for cataracts. It is called by one authority "One-day surgery for cataracts". It is claimed that the use of these new instruments will reduce the heavy medical and surgical costs because it will allow the patient to return to work the day after surgery.

"Two of these newer devices are built around a hollow needle. In one, the needle contains a tiny whirling blade that works like a Waring blender to pulverize the lens, which is then drawn off through a tube by a miniature Archimedes-screw pump. In the other device, the needle vibrates like a pneumatic drill, but at an ultrasonic

40,000 beats per second. A sensitive system emits fluid to flush away the lens debris.

"Eye surgeons at the famed Cleveland Clinic have started experimenting on rabbits with the 'blender', which was developed at the nearby Lewis Research Center of the National Aeronautics & Space Administration. Meanwhile, eye doctors are keenly watching the results of operations already being performed in eight U.S. hospitals with the 'ultrasonic' instruments, which are made by Cavitron Corp. in Santa Ana, Calif.

"This blending device is the creation of Cleveland's ophthalmologist Dr. William J. McGannon, who donated his idea for it to the NASA center two years ago, after working on it in his own comparatively inadequate research facilities for five years. Two NASA scientists, Donald J. Vargo and Dr. John C. Evvard, applied agency technical knowhow to perfecting it. Vargo, Evvard and McGannon are listed as co-inventors in a patent application. However, NASA, by its own policy, will assume all rights to the device and license it free to all comers.

Here is another method.

"Cavitron's ultrasonic device, called a Phaco Emulsifier, was invented by Dr. Charles D. Kelman, a New York ophthalmologist, who assigned his rights to the company. Kelman says the instrument's fluid control system, though adding to cost, is designed to avoid damage to eye structures.

"With both devices, only a 1/10-in. slit in the eye's transparent cornea is needed to get at the lens, in contrast to the 3/4-in. slit used in conventional surgery. The smaller incision can be closed by a single suture, and this heals faster than the larger opening. It is also less likely to be jarred open accidentally.

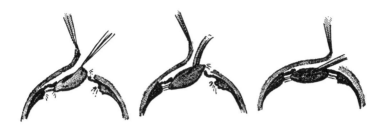

CATARACTS were once removed with forceps (above left) through a 180-degree incision (below left). The cryogenic probe (above center) now used by most surgeons requires a large incision, but Kelman's technique (above right) leaves only a single suture (below right).

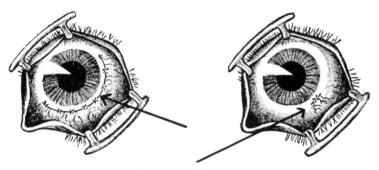

Cataract Surgery

"Not all doctors are sold on ultrasonics for cataract surgery. One reason, which Kelman stresses, rests with conventional surgery's enviable record of restoring vision. Though Kelman has used a Phaco Emulsifier to operate on 350 patients at Manhattan Eye, Ear & Throat Hospital over the past four years, other surgeons feel the technique is less proven than what they have been using.

"Another reason for reluctance is given by Dr. John S. Kennerdell, assistant professor of ophthalmology and neurology at the University of Pittsburgh, who has been operating with a Phaco Emulsifier at Pittsburgh's Eye & Ear Hospital since the ultrasonic instrument was installed there early this year. He says the emulsifier's delicacy and complexity discourage surgeons already skilled in conventional cataract procedures. Still, acceptance of ultrasonics is picking up. Kelman this year trained 26 surgeons to use the emulsifier, and it has been used in about 600 operations so far."

Such is progress in cataract surgery and no doubt there will be more . . . much more, to come in the near future.

I have deliberately given great detail in this chapter so that (a) you will know the many and varied versions of cataract surgery, (b) so that you will know that all is not as simple as some would have you believe, (c) so that you will be able to make a proper decision as to whether you want surgery or try natural methods to correct the condition, (d) so that you will understand that while the 'extraction of the lens' is successfully performed, your vision may not be all that is promised or desired.

10 After Cataract Surgery

Frequently we hear statements coming from the medical experts to the effect that . . . once we have cataract or glaucoma there is nothing to be done but surgery.

One worker who has helped thousands with their cataract conditions by only natural means makes this statement "I've helped children 18 months old and I've helped men in their 97th year." This practitioner claims that all sufferers of these conditions should not give up hope. Naturally there is much greater promise for those who catch the condition at an early stage. Surgery is by no means the answer. Surgery is used so frequently because it is the easiest way out. It shifts the responsibility from the individual to the healer and that's what everybody is looking for today . . . to shift responsibility, even if it results in blindness.

I wish sincerely that I could say that cataract surgery is the answer to cataract. My stand regarding surgery in general is well known. I am entirely opposed to the general use of surgery in the health of mankind. In cases of accident and various emergencies and such there may be justification for surgery. So I make no bones about it. I do not feel that surgery is the boon to mankind that the surgical profession and others make it appear to be. But in spite of the way I feel I have to admit that at least two forms of widely practised surgery have proven of tremendous benefit and value to mankind. First and foremost, is surgery for hernia and secondly, surgery for the prostate problem. No doubt there are other types of diseases and sicknesses that require surgery but I only cite those with which I am familiar. Therefore, when I claim that surgery for cataract is unwarranted or unnecessary I say this after taking into consideration all the facts that I have examined concerning cataracts.

To state that I inexorably oppose the use of surgery in cataract would not be the truth. When cataracts have been permitted to go their full scope and people will not or cannot follow a natural way of life with a drastic change in diet, which could relieve or correct the condition, then by all means surgery is in order and totally and fully warranted. After all, if a person is afflicted with fully developed cataract he is practically blind and therefore any means of assisting or aiding this condition is justified. In these cases I'm all for surgery even though these people have to wear the glasses with the built-in lenses. But by having the surgery and wearing these glasses at least they can see and find their way about.

However, I do feel that every possible means or method which is not harmful or injurious should be tried to correct the condition and produce some results. If I were afflicted with cataract I would not try any means that might possibly do more damage and cause a worse condition than I already had so I would be most selective in what I tried to do to correct the condition. I would have no hesitation in trying the cineraria maritima, the concentrated food supplements, urine therapy, honey and the linseed oil treatment, the sea water treatment and the eye exercises. Those I would unhesitatingly experiment with before submitting to surgery and I certainly and definitely would try the raw food diet first and foremost. I would also be willing to try the herbal methods because I have known for many long years that herbs seldom, if ever, do injury.

Let me quote from a researcher who has been doing work to improve defective sight for many, many years.

"Today, practically all the medical experts, from the American Medical Association to the distinguished eye specialist, to the general practitioner, will tell you there is only one satisfactory approach to the problem of cataract: diagnose, let it develop, operate. In most cases the second eye is affected as well. The usual procedure is to operate to remove the crystalline lens from the more affected eye, then later, at what is considered the proper time, the second eye is operated on in its turn. Then usually a series of heavy cataract lenses are fitted to replace the missing lens. These glasses have to be worn for the rest of the patient's life. Without them he is blind.

"Doctors will tell you that after the operation the sight is never as good as with the normal eye. In time, after the operation (if it is 'successful'), the vision straight ahead through the glasses is comparatively satisfactory, but the side vision is said to be lost."

I have written and sought information from people who have had surgery asking that they tell me just what their experience has been so that I could pass this information on to my readers. First let me start off by quoting a letter which I read in the Journal of The American Medical Association. This is in reply to an article by Dr. David Lester Ph.D., of Buffalo, in which he asked the readers of the Journal if any of them knew of any data relevant to the problem (suicide).

"From this letter in the journal seven U.S. doctors replied, all of whom had had personal experience about such behavior or who were able to cite authors who had written on the subject. One physician cited the case of an old farmer who jumped to his death four days after an operation for removal of cataracts. A New York physician reported two patients who had attempted suicide after successful cataract removal. Also, this same doctor claimed he had several other patients who showed post-operative anxiety, depression and withdrawal.

"Another cited the case history of a 52-year-old patient who committed suicide within a year after restoration of sight.

"Another physician reported that he had found many patients who became distressed after their sight was restored. They mentioned one patient who complained, 'How comes it that I now find myself less happy than before? Everything that I see causes me a disagreeable emotion. Oh, I was much more at ease in my blindness!' "

I have one rather pertinent comment to make on this situation. Most people who wait to have cataract surgery and then go through the agony of having the surgery, expect when all is O.K. with the surgery and the bandage is removed that they will be able to see again. Then what a great disappointment it is to go through this whole rigamarole and then wind up as though you were looking through a thick haze and never really see again without glasses as long as you live because cataract surgery removes your lens and never again is vision remotely what it was. What I'm trying to say is that they expect and are promised what they can never hope to achieve and thus the depression and often the suicide.

It must be remembered that a successful cataract operation means only that the 'lens of the eye has been successfully removed'. Since when does the mutilation of an organ constitute 'success'?

SURGERY . . . GOOD OR BAD?

Here I am quoting a group of letters. I made no attempt to influence anyone. Some are delighted with the results of surgery and others are deeply disappointed. Therefore, it is entirely up to the individual to appraise the situation in its true light and make his own decision.

The only suggestion that I have to offer is that common sense indicates that before resorting to 'irreversible, forever-gone surgery' you owe it to yourself to try one or more of the comparatively simple and harmless methods. Do not permit yourself to be rushed into irretractable surgery. At least inform yourself on as many aspects as possible. Discuss the matter with your loved ones and those concerned and then make your decision.

Here is a very interesting letter, especially since it deals with one of the newest and most advanced surgical techniques in cataract surgery.

"On advice of my doctor I waited as long as possible before having surgery on my eyes. I did this because they said there was always a possibility of losing your eyesight; so go as long as you can. I did just that, so I was near blind at the time of my operation.

"I had Dr. Bell here at Seneca call Dr. Kelman's office and they were very nice to me. They gave me my first appointment in New York for an examination; not surgery, just an examination. The examination was in May, 1971, then my appointment for surgery was the following September, 1971.

"I went to Dr. Kelman's office and they checked my eyes again at their clinic, then checked me in the Manhattan Eye, Ear and Throat Hospital; that was about noon. They started giving what medication they thought I needed that afternoon and night. The very next morning, at 9:30 A.M., I went in for surgery and in about, I would say, 45 minutes I was back in my room. They gave me something with a needle in my arm to put me to sleep, and I mean sound asleep as I did not know anything until it was all over. I became a little sick after I returned to my room, but they gave me a shot in the arm and that ended that. I had a patch over my eye with a Protectine shield. There was just nothing to it.

"It was just that simple. The very next morning they took the shield off my eye about 9:30 A.M. They looked at my eye and said go home. Well, I checked out of the hospital very shortly and went back across the street to Dr. Kelman's office for an examination before departure homeward.

"I came home on the plane by myself; no patch on my eye or glasses, except sun shades. My wife met me this time at the Greenville-Spartanburg Airport and brought me home. I went back to work in my restaurant the next day.

"Well in a very few days Dr. Bell fitted that eye with the thick lens type glasses. Man, I could not believe the world could be so bright.

"Then, I had my second appointment for surgery Dec. 26, 1971. It was the same routine; checked in and had surgery the next morning. At 9:30 check out, the next morning at 9:30 I went by Dr. Kelman's office for a check-up, then to airport and home. Remember I am always by myself.

"Dr. C. R. Duncan is my follow up specialist

(Ophthalmologist) at the Greenville, S.C. Carolina Eye Associates. Dr. Duncan said Dr. Kelman did a wonderful job. He called in another ophthalmologist who works in the same building (Dr. Jervis) who said it was great, and was a beautiful job.

"Well, let's talk a little about the results. I went for a check-up at Dr. Duncan's office Jan. 15th on a Monday. He said my eyes were fine and doing great. I had a 20-20 vision. This is the first time I have gone for a check-up in about 9 months.

"I am still wearing thick glasses with no contact lens at all. I am planning on contact lenses in the near future."

Here is another letter from a reader.

"I have been told that I had an excellent eye surgeon; usually there is a distortion of the pupil known as a keyhole, rather than that I have what looks like a small extra pupil above my natural one. After normal hospital tests, I went to surgery, using local anesthetic, at 10 A.M., was sitting up on my bed eating dinner at noon. No after effects, a laxative so I wouldn't strain, orders not to let my head get below my knees. A patch, eye drops periodically. Three days later, patch off, thick, heavy dark glasses. Vision immediately, distorted, but colors much brighter than before, spectacular. Through those glasses things and people are big, walking down a corridor I want to pass with a foot of clearance — more likely to make it 3-4 feet, resulting in running into the opposite wall. Released to go home a week after surgery, the only restriction, 'Don't get hit in that eye!' I have to use atropine during the healing process, this opens the pupil so that in bright sunlight too much gets in, the eye hurts. Use black patch. Vision better and better as the site of the operation healed. For glasses, one thick and one normal lens, one eye still not operated on. They don't work together. Things look larger and

117

brighter with the operated eye. Brighter, because the natural lens cuts down some light, and it is no longer there. As long as I have an unoperated eye to compare against I'm afraid of using the operated eye, distance judgement is not so good, stairs and curbstones present problems. I have a device to block either eye. Without either eye being blocked I would see two of whatever I looked at, one large, one smaller. Turn my head and the position of the larger would change. When some part of the object matched in both images, the operated eye would take over, and the unoperated eye just wouldn't register its image in my brain, the other is brighter. After a little practice I found that by an effort of will I could use either eye, disregarding the image from the other entirely.

"A contact lens would make the eyes work together, for the contact lens so near the location of the original would produce an image only very slightly larger, the brain would fuse them together automatically. Fine, when it worked, and the 3D vision was spectacular. But I got 'flare', making lights have something like part of a peacock's tail shooting out SW and NE. Also, the lens generated a small ulcer on the cornea. With surgery on the other inevitable, I abandoned contacts for the time.

"One thing proven: the Bates theory of accommodation for distances is wrong.* Only the lens was removed. None of the muscles Bates says are used were touched. Thus I should have the same accommodation I had before surgery, accommodation equal to that of the unoperated eye. And I have none at all. With the far section of the spectacle lens vision is good from 5-6 feet to the far distance, perhaps clearest at 50-60 feet, but very good indeed at greater distances. With the contact lens alone this might be from 3-4 feet to the far distance,

* I feel this patient was in no position to judge because his eye did not have sufficient time to adjust to the drastic change and with the two different conditions and focus of the eyes he could not judge the power of accommodation.

118

peaking around 100 feet. With the bifocal section of the spectacles, or using the contact plus my old glasses, there is a definite distance around 15-16 inches where vision is very clear. Two to three inches one way or the other it is usable, but just a trifle fuzzy. It is evident that Bates was wrong on that score.

"Final results: After the second eye was operated on and I had to use the cataract glasses, and had no standard for comparison, I rapidly got used to them. To the complete amazement of my ophthalmologist, my optometrist was able to predict the prescription for the second eye accurately, from his knowledge of its previous requirements, and the effect of surgery on the first eye. Vision is now dependably 20-20, often 20-15 or better. The distance of the chart is a factor, usually it is not quite in focus for the distant section, but moving the glasses out about 1/16 inch will bring it in. My TV screen is too far away for the near section, too close for the distant section. Move the glasses about 1/8 inch out — I can count the scanning lines on the screen! Push the glasses toward my eyes a little, and I can read that sign so distant that others cannot."

This is a letter from a friend of mine.

"Because I, too, want to be of assistance to others I shall give you details about my cataract surgery. If, after you read this, there is more you desire, please write and I shall try to comply with your request.

"Dr. Robert Lehner of Racine, Wisc. did my surgery on Monday, December 20 at St. Mary's Hospital in Racine. I came back from the recovery room about 4 in the afternoon, the surgery had been done at 7:30 a.m. I was very uncomfortable all that evening because of a back ache and having to pass water so frequently. My eye did not bother me at all.

"On Tuesday, the day after surgery, I walked about and fed myself. I returned to the convent on Thursday and attended Christmas Eve Mass on Saturday the 25th.

"I am Treasurer of our Community . . . the Monday after I had surgery our nurse allowed me to work in my office one hour in the morning and one hour in the afternoon. I remained in our convent infirmary for 2 weeks.

"I work part time as a broker in Milwaukee and after a 3-week leave of absence I returned to work. I had to wear a patch over the eye for about 6 weeks and during this time I did not drive. As soon as the patch came off for good I drove my car again.

"When the eye stabilized, they checked my vision and it was like a miracle as I could read 20/30 vision. However, that was short lived. By the time the large, thick, lens came and later when the contact lens came I could not read at all. Something had happened.

"The man who was working with me on the contact lens, Richard Mickschl of Milwaukee, had tried both the hard lens and the soft lens; neither worked and he suggested that I see another doctor. He recommended the men who handle problem cases at the Milwaukee County General Hospital. The 10th floor is devoted to diseases of the eye.

"My original doctor had to recommend me and he did. I first saw Dr. Robert A. Hyndiuk who specializes in cornea work. He and 3 other men gave me a 3-hour examination. They felt a cornea transplant would do the trick, but wanted Dr. Thomas M. Aaberg to see me as they thought they saw an ulcer on the retina. After I saw him this was his report: a) Fluid had collected on the retina; this happens in about 2% of cataract patient cases. There is about a 50% chance that the fluid will go away. There is no cure for it . . . no medication, no shots, no surgery. b) Not to have cataract surgery in the other eye as most likely the fluid would collect there too. c) If the fluid goes away of its own accord it usually does so within 3 months after surgery.

"After all these examinations I returned to my original doctor and he had the report from the two specialists. He said he had the fluid experience with his sister-in-law and hers disappeared after about a year; also he had to do surgery on the 2nd eye and she did not have the same sad experience with it.

"That is where I am now. I am praying that the fluid will leave, but that is in the hands of God. In the meantime I get along as well as I can. I am still doing the work of the Treasurer and also working 3 days a week as a broker . . . not any less than I did before, but it is so difficult. However, people are so good. Knowing of my blindness, they are most helpful.

"Whatever you can do for cataract patients will surely be a blessing for it is a difficult period to adjust to. — Sister J. E. M."

The following is a letter from a reader-subscriber.

"Dear Sir, — I do thank you for asking me to write you for that is what I have wanted to do for some time. I wanted to ask what you think of my condition and what I can do to be myself again.

"Two years ago I had an operation on my right eye for cataract. Before the operation the doctor told me that I would be unable to keep my balance, or rather that I would stagger in walking for some time but I would get over it in about six or eight months.

"It has been two years now and I am yet staggering. If the surface is smooth I do fairly well, but the slightest roughness nearly throws me down. I forgot to tell you I am 78 years old, but they say I don't look it. I don't think so myself unless you see me walk. Then I think I walk like someone over 90.

"Pray tell me what I can do to remedy this condition. The doctor does not know."

Here is another reader's cataract surgery experience.

"About my cataract surgery, there is really not too much to tell. In my middle forties my eyesight began to dim so I went to an eye specialist and he told me I had a cataract pretty well developed on one eye and another one started on the other eye. Believe me, this was an awful blow to have this condition when I was so young. Anyway, the cataracts continued to develop and I had eye surgery (removal of the lens) on March 1953 and August 1953. I have worn cataract glasses ever since.

"Of course these cataract lenses are my eyes now. I have pretty good vision with the glasses but can't see without them. I don't have good side vision but I do get along pretty well. I have two brothers and two sisters who have also had the same operation. My mother had cataracts so I am sure it is a hereditary trait that runs in the family on my mother's side."

Here we have a rather disappointing experience.

"You asked if anyone knew of a successful treatment or cure for cataracts. Sure do wish that I'd known of one 4 years ago, was nearly blind before I 'broke down' and went to the VA Hospital. They cut one out and the other 18 days later. Have to wear thick, heavy glasses . . . can't see my big nose without them."

In the uniocular surgery the ophthalmologist and the surgeon usually advise contact lenses so that the super-powered spectacle lenses need not be worn but so far the contact lens to correct this problem has not been proven 100% successful.

Broadly speaking, the basic surgical procedure concerning cataracts remains the same as it has been for many years. However, cryosurgery is being used and the medical profession claims that it does facilitate the removal of the lens from behind the iris. The reason for the cryosurgery is that in many instances it can lessen the possibility of rupturing the capsule during the removal of the lens.

According to the best medical authority if all the crystalline lens has been removed, the cataract will never return. However, if the capsule has ruptured and portions of the lens remain in the eye, these remnants can become more opaque and a second operation may be needed.

When the crystalline lens is removed it creates a refractive deficiency making the affected eye extremely farsighted. For this reason extra power spectacle lenses must be used to correct the deficiency and enable the individual to see properly once again. Due to the positioning of the spectacle lens some distance from the crystalline lens's former position inside the eye, a sizable amount of retinal image magnification usually occurs. In the binocular surgery the extra magnification is not a weighty problem because both eyes are affected and you just understand that everything looks much bigger than normal and you soon adapt to your new eyes, so to speak. However, with the uniocular surgery it is absolutely impossible for both eyes to function simultaneously . . . at least not without incurring double vision. This is what I meant when I said it creates a traumatic situation when you have to have one eye operated on at a time.

A glass spectacle lens correcting the natural lens to focus light on the retinal layer of the eye.

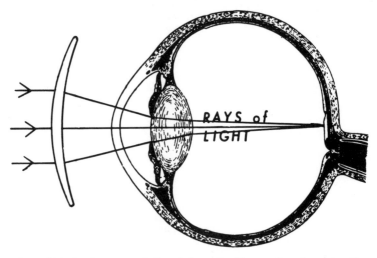

RAYS of LIGHT

The slightly increased focal length (from the lens to the retina of the eye) still permits wide angle viewing and maintains normal image size.

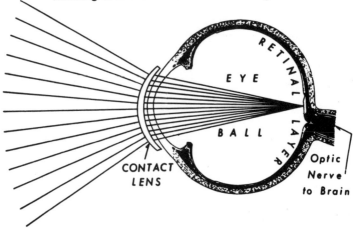

EYE BALL

RETINAL LAYER

CONTACT LENS

Optic Nerve to Brain

I hold in my hand a volume published in 1847 and written by William White Cooper, Fellow of the Royal College of Surgeons of England; fellow of the Royal Medical and Chirurgical Society; senior surgeon to the

North London Ophthalmic Institution, and to the Honourable Artillery Company; surgeon to the School For Teaching the Blind, etc. The book is entitled "Practical Remarks On Near Sight, Aged Sight, And Impaired Vision; with observations upon the use of glasses and on artificial light."

You may ask of what relevance is a book over 125 years old. So I say to you ... don't judge until you have read the quotations that I have extracted from the book, then judge their merit.

"Cataract Glasses — The object aimed at in operations for cataract, is either to extract the opaque crystalline lens from the eye; to cause its absorption; or to displace it so as to give a free passage to light. As the image formed on the retina depends upon the refractions produced by means of the crystalline lens and on its power of self adjustment to objects at different distances, the consequences of its loss usually are, indistinctness of vision and loss of power of accommodation to distance. If, prior to the formation of cataract, the eye was perfect (not merely as to its power to define objects at a given distance, but as to the power of adjustment to distance also), there is after the operation an incapability of discerning near objects, as the eye no longer has the power to accommodate itself to the necessary focus.

"To remedy these inconveniences double convex glasses are employed;* and it is necessary to have two pairs,

* The lenses used by divers, if made of crown glass and equiconvex, must have the curvatures of both surfaces equal to that of the cornea, for in order that the refraction of such a lens may be equal to that of the cornea which it is intended to supply, the focal length of the lens in water, must be equal to that of the cornea in air.

It must be borne in mind that when the eye is immersed in water, the first and most considerable of its refractions is lost, for the refractive power of the aqueous humour is very nearly that of water, and so the cornea being bounded by surfaces which are nearly parallel, the rays will pass from water into the aqueous humour without undergoing refraction. Thus a powerful convex lens is required to afford distinct vision.

of different focal lengths; one for looking at distant objects, the other for reading and writing.

"A cataract glass should, when placed in front of the eye, give perfect vision of objects at the distance at which they could be distinctly seen before the change in the lens commenced. If the focus is too long, the patient will find it necessary after a time to remove the glasses two or three inches from the eyes in order to see distinctly: in such a case glasses of a shorter focus must be procured. If the focus is too short, the patient will mistake the distance of objects from him, as they will appear nearer than they really are, and the hand, in the effort to grasp them, will fall short of them.

"For some time after operation for cataract, the patient, (especially if young), should endeavour to do as much as possible without glasses, for although *the adjusting power inherent in the eye is destroyed by the operation,* nature will, if compelled, make great efforts to provide a substitute. Mr. Middlemore observes, ** 'Some years ago I operated on a child four years old, and directed the little patient's friends not to employ glasses to assist his sight, without my permission: they carefully obeyed my directions, and this boy is not at the present time much more far-sighted than many persons whose lens has not been removed.'

"Sir. W. Adams operated upon a postillion who was blind from cataract in both eyes. When the man resumed his employment he wore spectacles, not being able even to walk without them: finding, however, that travellers objected to be driven by a person requiring spectacles, he gradually left them off, and at the end of twelve months could drive and walk perfectly well without their aid.

** A Treatise on the Diseases of the Eye. Vo. ii. p. 202.

"Glasses, then, should not under any circumstances be permitted for a considerable time after the operation, nor indeed so long as vision continues to improve without them. If they be used too early, and the glasses are too powerful, the eyes may become enfeebled and require more and more assistance, so that after a time no lenses will be found of sufficient power. If the individual will wait until the eye has completely recovered, and will habituate the organ as much as possible to its altered state, he will then be in a condition to select glasses of a proper strength, and these if used sparingly, will probably serve him all his life."

"I have known an instance of imperfect congenital cataract that was for many years mistaken for aggravated myopia.

" Case I. — 'The patient, a gentleman of thirty years of age, in consulting me respecting his sight, states, that he has been exceedingly nearsighted from childhood, and acting under the advice of a medical man, he has for some time worn double concave glasses, but without deriving benefit — that his sight is decidedly getting worse. Upon his attempting to read tolerably large type, he holds the book very near to his eyes and turns his back to the window, that at the same time he may illuminate the object and keep his eyes in the shade. It is with difficulty he makes out even a few words, saying that the letters appear confused and misty. On examining the pupils when under the influence of light, I find them contracted to the size of mere pinholes; small however as the pupil is, beyond it I perceive something grey. To ascertain the nature of this, I put the eyes under the influence of atropine, and then have a distinct view of a cataract, greyish and jelly-like, obstructing the central portion of each pupil, but allowing while the pupils are dilated, of the access of light all around. Through this space, my patient for the first time in his life sees distinctly. All objects appear to him to have undergone a transformation as if they had been touched

127

with a magician's wand. Upon looking at a mirror, he discovers for the first time that his eyes are blue. Colours appear immeasurably brighter than he had ever imagined, and though the day is cloudy, he expressed much surprise at the brightness of the light. The glory of the sun he has yet to see. This morning he first discerns the features of the members of his family, and it is highly interesting, and not a little touching, to observe his feelings, and the surprise he envinces at the erroneous impressions which he had formed, for as he observes, 'Until now I have never seen like other people.' It is a satisfaction to me to be able to state, that by a very trifling operation his newly-acquired powers of vision have been rendered permanent.' "

It is interesting to note that atropine was used then (1847) and it is still used today in 1973.

"The period of life at which presbyopia displays itself, is the same as that at which hard cataract commences; and it is possible that the imperfection of vision, arising from the commencement of hard cataract, may be confounded with presbyopia, by one who is not familiar with ophthalmic diseases.

"A decided opinion as to the non-existence of cataract can only be ventured on with safety, after the pupil has been dilated with belladonna. When cataract does exist, it will generally be seen on dilating the pupil fully, as a greenish, grayish, or amber-coloured haze in the centre of the pupil; and of an opacity in proportion as the nucleus is hard. It is by no means unusual, when the iris is under the influence of this valuable drug, to find spots in the lens, or streaks extending from the circumference towards the centre; or even the whole margin of the lens opaque. Yet these changes will be concealed by the iris if the pupil is in its natural condition: much credit has at times been gained for superior skill in the detection of cataract by simple attention to this one point.

128

"Dilatation of the pupil is effected most rapidly, and for the longest time, by dropping into the eye a solution of the neutral sulphate of atropine,* in the proportion of two or four grains to the ounce of distilled water. A full drop placed in the eye by means of a camel's hair pencil produces no pain. The lids should be closed for ten minutes, and the effect is usually produced in from fifteen to twenty minutes. I have known the pupil to remain under the influence of one application for eleven days. It should be borne in mind, that the preparations of belladonna have the effect of depriving the eye, for a time, of a portion of its power of adjustment. It is found that, as the dilatation of the pupil increases, the point of distinct vision is removed further from the eye. The inconvenience is, however, but temporary, but it is well that the patient should be warned of this effect, lest he imagine that the eye has been injured by the application of the belladonna."

From my correspondence and investigations I have found that the later the special cataract lenses are prescribed the greater the chance of improvement due to the eye accommodating itself by various natural bodily adjustments. This, along with the evidence presented in William White Cooper's book, sort of blasts into smithereens the Helmholtz theory that accommodation is accomplished solely by the various actions of the lens. Also, it supports Dr. Bates' findings that the eye itself plays a role in accommodation.

* That which I use is prepared by Mr. Bullock, of Conduit Street. I have some in my possession which was prepared early in 1844, and it is yet perfectly good.

129

11 Contact Lenses

I am going to give you a broad picture of the contact lens story from various contact lens manufacturers and medical authorities.

Let me quote from several authoritative sources. This happens to be from one of the foremost manufacturers or producers of contact lens.

"All modern contact lenses are thin plastic disks which fit either over the entire visible portion of the eye (scleral lenses) or over the pupil and iris area (corneal lenses). They are optically prescribed and ground on the outer side to correct or improve your vision — while the inner side is carefully prescribed and designed to correspond to the surface shape of your eye. All lenses hold a thin layer of liquid against the cornea. In conventional scleral lenses this liquid is a special chemical solution. Corneal lenses and ventilated scleral lenses utilize the wearer's natural tears instead of the chemical solution.

"Corneal lenses, about half the size of a dime, actually

131

float on the eye's natural layer of tears. They are held in place by capillary attraction. Scleral lenses fit under the eyelids and rest evenly on the white portion of the eyes.

"Once learned, the insertion and removal of contact lenses is very simple. A lens is removed by a tug at the corner of the eye while the eye is wide open. It is inserted by being brought up to the eye on the finger tip and blinked into place. Contact lens can be thought of as eyeglasses that are worn directly on the eyes instead of half an inch in front of them. The difference between placing a lens on the eye and placing it slightly in front may seem minor, hardly worth the time, thought, and effort expended in the development of contact lenses during the past century and a half.

"Contact lenses, in a sense, become a part of the eye itself, unlike spectacles, which are really windowpanes that the eyes look through. Just like eyes themselves, contact lenses cannot steam up or become streaked in the rain.

"To remove a corneal lens the head is bent forward and the eyes are opened as wide as possible without the aid of fingers. A slightly upward pull at the outer corner of the eye releases the lens. The lens then drops into the outstretched hand.

"About nine people out of ten can safely switch from spectacles to contact lenses. But can does not necessarily mean should.

"Widely advertised claims that anybody can wear contact lenses with comfort, almost immediately, are entirely false! The lens is a foreign body when placed on the eye. Time and patience are needed to overcome one's instinctive fear of inserting the lenses and to develop a tolerance for wearing them.

"Successful adjustment to contact lenses depends largely on one's own mental attitude toward them Determination is required to wear them every day for increasingly long periods of time and to persevere in practicing their insertion and removal. Some people can wear contact lenses with complete comfort after only a few days. Others may require several weeks. A few may have so strong a psychological block that they can never wear them.

"Of course, contact lenses can be worn safely and comfortably only when the fit is perfect. They are not mere mechanical gadgets. They become, in effect, part of a delicate, sensitive organ — the human eye. Only a trained professional is qualified to fit them."

CONTACT LENS DON'T'S

1. Don't rub your eyes with the lenses on.

2. Don't sleep with your lenses on.

3. Don't demonstrate with your lenses around other people.

4. Don't let others handle or use your lenses.

5. Don't step if you drop a lens, look for it first.

6. Don't go swimming with your lenses on, unless you have your doctor's permission.

7. Don't expect to wear or be comfortable with the lenses when you are ill or in the hospital. Check with your doctor about a wearing schedule.

8. If you have broken your wearing schedule, do not resume your schedule where you left off. You will probably have to back off a bit

on your schedule and should check with your doctor for proper instructions.

9. Contact lenses are expensive and rather easy to lose. Be sure you know what replacement lenses would cost and whether or not you have some type of loss coverage. Don't guess at what your replacement policy does for you. Read and know it well.

10. The welfare of your eyes and lenses depends upon careful examination at specific intervals. Don't miss your appointments and always let your doctor know when the lenses are uncomfortable.

"It is claimed that the need to change contact lenses is much less frequent than with eyeglasses. They state that lenses should be carefully handled to prevent scratching, chipping, cracking or breaking. Wearers with long fingernails should be especially careful in handling the lenses."

Now I'd like to quote this from another publication put out by a leading optical firm. "His practitioner may prescribe or recommend a contact lens as the preferred solution for the individual need. Whether he does or not, the patient will undoubtedly require a pair of glasses for reading and for those occasions when his contact lenses are not readily available or are out of use."

ARE CONTACT LENSES DIFFICULT TO USE?

"The answer is no, but here again this must be qualified by pointing out that each patient's visual needs are unique. Therefore, each person's type of problem and his determination to enjoy the advantages offered by contact lenses will determine how easily he learns to handle, care for, and wear contact lenses.

"Each experienced patient, whether he is in kindergarten or in his seventies, can apply or remove a contact lens simply and painlessly. But a new wearer must have patience, because this wonderful aid to vision is at first a stranger to the eye — no matter how carefully and correctly it is prescribed and adjusted. The beginner will gradually learn to accept this stranger — just as one must learn to wear other prosthetic devices comfortably.

"This 'adaptation period' will vary: it may mean weeks or months for one patient, and much longer for another. Your optometrist will make frequent inspections of your eyes as well as the lenses and custom fit during this period to make certain that everything is proceeding according to plan. When it eventually arrives, 'comfort' is a varying degree of unconsciousness to the presence of these small lenses on the eyes. After adaptation to a set of properly prescribed and adjusted contact lenses, you can generally expect to wear them comfortably and without fear of damage to your eyes for long periods, possibly up to the full waking day."

Here is a quote from Herald of Health, October 1966.

"Contact Lens Danger — A research team at the Corneal Centre, New York, reports in the British Medical Journal of January 15, 1966, that contact lenses permit only about 1/100 of the necessary oxygen to the cornea of the eye. These lenses inhibit the flow of the tear fluid on the corneal surface — the only source and channel of oxygen supply to the tissues of the eye. This may lead to atrophy of the tissues which may eventually become cancerous."

I'd like to report some of the goings on from the Canadian Ophthalmological Society Meeting at Harrison Hot Springs, B.C., in September, 1972. "Three consecutive papers which were represented at the meeting described

135

complications that were found in hydrophilic lenses, ranging from mysterious disintegration of the plastic in some patients' eyes to strange fungal growths which seem to digest the plastic, and abrasive particles left on the lenses through poor quality controls at the manufacturing end."

"There are two major manufacturers of contact lens and one of these companies came in for rather outspoken criticism due to the frequency of changes in design as well as the formulation of storage solutions and poor quality control on its lathe-turned lenses, which resulted in polymer plastic debris which in turn causes eye irritation.

"The chief ophthalmologist at Scarborough General Hospital, Dr. Harold Stein, presented one of the largest assessments of soft contact lenses to date — 405 eyes in 213 patients since February 1971. The great majority (375 lenses) were fitted for cosmetic reasons, and Dr. Stein confined his report to these patients.

"Both the Griffin lens and the competitive Bausch & Lomb lens were fitted, chosen 'on the basis of their chronological availability' as Dr. Stein put it. The patients were selected because of their desire to wear contacts, plus their suitability. Of the 375 lenses fitted, 182 were Griffin, and it was here that the first criticism of this manufacturer emerged.

" 'Assessment was difficult because the manufacturer has made many changes in lens design and the formulation of sterilization and storage solutions,' said Dr. Stein. 'As a result, the patients suffered a credibility gap which had a psychological effect on their continued use of the lens.' In fact, the Griffin group in Dr. Stein's series suffered a 37% failure rate, with poor vision given as the major cause."

Please note "A 37% failure rate, with poor vision given as the major cause". "There were 131 replacements in

136

all for reasons of breakage or poor vision." "By contrast, the 146 patients fitted with Bausch & Lomb lenses had a 16% failure rate — with poor fluctuating vision as the main cause. Although there was some irritation of the eye, there was no conjunctivitis, and a high percentage of the patients reported vision equal to that with spectacles. 'We found that when we tried some of the patients who had failed with the Griffin lenses — most of whom had had trouble with chipping and replacement — they were happily fitted with the Bausch & Lomb lenses', said Dr. Stein."

The following is Dr. Stein's summation of the advantages and disadvantages of soft contact lenses.

ADVANTAGES

1. Comfort: within 30 min. the patient hardly knows he is wearing them.

2. Interchangeable with spectacles, and can be worn intermittently for athletic or social events.

3. Minimal lens loss, since they adhere strongly to the eye.

4. Minimal overwear reaction.

5. Lack of glare and photophobia. The soft lenses seem to have some absorptive quality of glare and ultraviolet.

DISADVANTAGES

1. The soft lenses mold to the eye and do not correct a significant amount of astigmatism (greater than one diopter).

2. Some patients complain of poor vision.

137

3. Chipping and poor quality control in one make of lens.

4. Poor vision may result from dehydration of the lens (corrected by immersing them in saline).

5. Modifications to the lens once it has been manufactured are impossible at present. A new lens is required if changes are required.

Here is another report headed: Red or Irritated Eyes Common In Wearers of Soft Contact Lenses.

"A New Westminster, B.C., ophthalmologist, Dr. Donald Johnson reports — Out of 200 patients fitted with Griffin soft contact lenses over an 18-month period, 120 returned at least once with a complaint of a red or irritated eye. Some of the reasons are: poor hygiene and improper use of solutions; wearing the lens inside out; wearing the lenses in opposite eyes; and crater-like erosions of the lens surface, apparently caused by fungus; and minute mounds of plastic material left behind by the manufacturer and missed in quality control checks at the plant.

"In addition, he confirmed reports by Dr. Stein that the Griffin lens was subject to splitting and tearing. 'This was an important problem in the early period,' added Dr. Johnson. 'It now seems to have been resolved and now appears to be largely the patient's fault'.

"Changes in the lens plastic caused the greatest number of cases of keratoconjunctivitis, and Dr. Johnson commented that usually the condition produced is among the most severe cases he has ever seen. 'There was marked conjunctival injection, edema, punctate epithelial erosion around the lens surface changes if they were on the posterior surface of the lens.' "

Here is what we are told by the contact lens specialists about contacts after surgery.

"For persons who experience difficulty in wearing corrective eyeglasses after cataract surgery, the use of the contact lens is increasing. These cornea-fitting lenses have several advantages. Thick cataract eyeglasses offer patients normal sight while they are looking straight ahead, but side vision is noticeably distorted. These glasses interfere with such activities as driving a car in which side vision is important. On the other hand, contact lenses grant patients the undistorted distant vision they had before the cataract, allowing them to perform any function where side vision is essential. A contact lens is often prescribed for patients who have had one cataract removed. The contact lens compensates for the difference in size of the image seen by the normal eye and by the eye operated on. Doctors have found that more than 75 per cent of the cataract patients for whom contact lens are prescribed learn to wear them successfully."

I would like to quote here the opinion of a qualified optometrist.

"To begin with, one must keep in mind that contact lenses are a 'foreign body' in contact with the cells of the body, known as corneal tissue. They are always tolerated, never accepted — as self.

"The firm (or what some call — 'hard') lenses on this basis cannot avoid interfering with cell function. The trick of the matter is to keep the interference below the capacity of the cells to tolerate and regenerate from the interference.

"What is the interference? One must understand that the cells forming the eyes are *BRAIN STUFF*. They have the same three specialized layers as the brain; in the case of brain the layers are called Dura mater, pia mater, arachnoid. Eyes — corneal, choroid and sclera.

"In the case of the eyes, we find living cells directly exposed to the cruel world. Nowhere else in the body is this the case. Think of the skin covering. And not only is theirs direct exposure to external reality, the cells so exposed are the *HIGHEST TYPE OF SPECIALIZED CELL VARIETY IN THE BODY*. They are the brain on display. This is why the multiple secretions of the lids and surrounding eye area pour out what is needed to keep the cells moist, nourished, cooled, oxidated . . . in short alive. And 16 hours per day for long years.

"When a contact of the firm type is put on the eye it interferes with all such activities. The eyes breathe, like the lungs do and this is interfered with. The tear flow is disturbed. The cells are scuffed, pressed upon (in some cases this is done intentionally so as to create a new profile and eliminate nearsightedness). A Toronto, Canada, optometrist has worked this out.

"But sleep and the marvelous capacity of the corneal cells to regenerate in just a few hours rest . . . restores the balance and the contact lenses can be tolerated. This tolerance is highest in the young female . . . age 12 thru 30. Eventually as circulation and other body functions decline, tolerance is lost and the contacts can no longer be worn successfully. This is why mature people are usually poor prospects. And at age 70 when circulation has declined some 80% . . . it's all over.

"To the question of 'permanent damage or injury' then, my belief is that none occurs in standard cases of proper wear. Something like an analogy of wearing shoes, which certainly soften the foot cells and make going barefooted a hazard for a few days but offer other benefits including protection against spine shock when the heel

140

(barefooted) hits the hard pavement.

"Of course for any knucklehead who gets drunk and wears the contacts three or four days straight . . . or longer for some other reason, as in being on drugs, anything can happen. One case I read about had them on two weeks and the lens sawed thru the conjunctiva and came to rest on the optic nerve. When it was discovered by a surgeon it had done a lot of damage.

"But in the usual case of good handling, wearing discipline the calculated risk involved is no more nor less than the probability factor associated with everything else in life. Driving the car, contending with falling asteroids, eating additives inadvertently, breathing contaminated air . . . all such life experiences have their own risk probability, i.e. 'threat to physical survival.' Since we are born to lose, no wonder Nietsche advised us to 'live dangerously.' (He meant embrace life dynamically, not smoke dynamite sticks).

"We know that the organized system labeled our body disorganizes inevitably. As Professor White (Harvard philosopher) commented on Jack Paar's show some years ago . . . to the viewing audience, says he: 'Remember you can't win.' So in this contacts aid the search for intervening happiness.

"My opinion therefore is that contact lenses, whether firm or soft variety are a useful tool for mankind to use when necessary. Proper use minimizes the potential hazard to an acceptable level. Improper use . . . well this is just as bad as smoking two packs a day. The Jackass factor will apparently always be with us."

Dr. R. O. Rychner, ophthalmologist at the National Medical Foundation for Eye Care in New York stated, "The use of contact lenses can at times lead to serious, permanent impairment of vision".

According to Capt. R. K. Lanshe, a Marine Corps eye specialist, "Corneal strangulation can result from wearing contact lenses with too sharp an inner curvature. This lens curve creates a suction-cup effect that can prevent the metabolic exchanges of gases, hypertonic tears, and heat."

Ophthalmologists quoted by Good Housekeeping (June, 1960) "Corneal abrasions are not uncommon. Though they heal quickly in most cases, you can get scarring and reduced vision. I tell all my patients that there is danger in wearing contact lenses."

From another article in Good Housekeeping we learn that "Certain people should never even try to wear contact lenses — diabetics; those with chronic colds or sinusitis; those with extra dry, teary, or abnormally protruding eyes." They warn against nicotine on the lenses; rubbing the eyes; or wearing lenses while eyes are irritated by colds, hay fever, or styes. Any one of these can cause a scratch on the cornea, which can lead to serious eye infection. Any break in the surface of the cornea gives germs a chance to enter, multiply, and cause infection. These can cause corneal scars that may reduce vision; worse, an ulcer may develop which, in some extensive cases, requires the eye's removal.

A routine sampling of 16 ophthalmologists across the United States brought out some startling facts: 15 of them had treated corneal injuries resulting from contact lenses, and 4 out of these had handled cases in which the eye was lost as a result of the damage.

ARE CONTACT LENSES DANGEROUS?

The following is the opinion of a leading optical association.

"Contact lenses are safe to wear, provided they are professionally prescribed, ground, and adjusted as well as properly used by the patient.

"The wearer needs to receive the close personal supervision of his optometrist during the adaptation period and then be certain to return for periodic checkups thereafter; this is to insure protection of the cornea, check the patient's care and use of the lenses and make minor adjustments if necessary.

"What happens if a patient is struck in the eye while wearing contact lenses? In the great majority of cases, the lens will do no damage to the eye — it may even act as a mechanical protector!

"In one of the many recorded cases, a contact lens wearer was thrown through a car windshield and her right eyelid was cut completely through in two places. Her contact lens had a deep scratch in it, but her eye was not damaged.

"When a contact lens is worn, blows to the eye tend to be distributed over a larger area; this affords greater protection to the wearer."

I must interject at this point . . . if you believe the above then you believe Grimm and Anderson wrote 'true stories'.

The following is further information from the optical companies.

ARE CONTACT LENSES
MORE EFFECTIVE THAN EYEGLASSES?

"Vision correction or improvement through any visual aid depends on the individual. Some visual problems can best be corrected or improved by wearing contact lenses, while success with other problems may require wearing eyeglasses (or perhaps both). Your optometrist can tell you whether contact lenses or eyeglasses will be more effective in treating your particular visual problems.

"Eligible contact lens wearers must consider various factors — good or bad — about contact lenses. The optometrist can help you decide whether the advantages plus your motivation to wear contact lenses outweigh the disadvantages in your case.

DISADVANTAGES

"Contact lenses require more care and can be misplaced easier than eyeglasses . . . they are relatively more expensive as well because extra hours of effort and additional skill are needed to provide safe and efficient results.

"A minimum of five or six office visits are required for prescribing and adjustments . . . although the total number of visits depends on the patient, the condition of his eyes, the type of lens used and the optometrist's judgement.

"Some visual problems cannot be corrected by contact lenses.

"Most people become more sensitive to light while wearing contact lenses.

"Successful adaptation cannot be guaranteed . . . some patients may achieve successful results only after 20 or more visits while others may never achieve satisfaction and comfort.

"Semi-annual evaluations are imperative following a

144

successful contact lens fitting to insure continued comfort, safety and efficiency.

ADVANTAGES

"Psychologically — many people do not like to wear glasses . . . with contact lenses they feel more socially well-adjusted because they look more attractive and gain confidence in themselves.

"Occupationally — dancers, models, singers and actors find them indispensable to their appearance and performance . . . surgeons like the lack of clouding from perspiration plus improved peripheral vision . . . those working with cameras, telescopes, microscopes or binoculars like the unobstructive convenience when viewing through their instruments . . . athletes appreciate the safety features . . . busy housewives like the stability of contact lenses for indoor-outdoor activity plus relief from the fashion-conscious necessity to match glasses with clothing.

"Optically — contact lenses allow a wider field of vision . . . present a less distorted and more realistic size of objects viewed . . . allow more efficient eyeteaming (ability of the eyes to work together) in some cases . . . are much better for extreme nearsightedness and often stop or slow its progression . . . do not 'fog' from rain or perspiration . . . can replace the thick, heavy eyeglass lenses needed by postoperative cataract patients . . . are a necessity and only solution for some types of eye defects and injuries . . . allow precision tolerances up to 1/400,000 of an inch . . . usually require changing less frequently than eyeglasses".

Now you've heard their side of the story.

Here is a quotation from the British Medical Journal, March 26, 1966: "Whatever its type or the material from which it is made, a contact lens must be considered a foreign body on the eye. Ideally, it should fit the anterior segment of the eye as a glove, be made of material that would alter its shape as does the eye, and allow respiration of the cornea and a free flow of tears either round the material or through it. In addition it must provide a fairly rigid front surface to correct the patient's vision. Such a lens should be wearable day and night without being removed and not be a source of contamination by virus, bacterium, or fungus to the eye and lids. Furthermore, the material must not undergo degenerative changes, with the production of toxic substances.

"Contact lenses with all these qualities have yet to be made."

Here I'll quote from the statement of a contact lens purchaser as it appeared in Consumer Bulletin (January, 1960). "At a contact lens specialist, I bought a pair of contact lenses. The standard price is, or was, $180.00. This, in my case included a pair of reading glasses to be worn with them and a bottle of liquid, which I was directed to use every time I used them. Because of the ever-present danger of losing the lenses by misplacement or having them fall out of the eye, I was advised to buy an insurance policy. Annual premium $15.00. ... I could see quite well with the lenses. There the satisfaction ended. Putting them in the eye requires the use of a special fluid, considerable skill and practice, a mirror and, preferably, privacy. ... Taking them out is another trick. ... This I know: Any talk about 'throwing away' your glasses is pure deception. You will need them.

"Having thought contact lenses primarily suited to outdoor activities, on boats (or swimming), my experience of losing them is just another time I was played for a sucker and should have known better. Nothing could be what the ads say contact lenses are. Fortunately, the

146

financial loss was not serious for me, but I do regret the evenings I spent with the cussed things in my eyes, crying copiously, looking down only, night after night."

It is known that one man some time ago in France contracted ulcers in both eyes because of contact lenses and he became completely blind. A St. Louis ophthalmologist writing in the American Journal of Ophthalmology, 12/65 stated that he had 12 patients whom he considered satisfied users of contact lenses, but suddenly all developed astigmatism. They quickly stopped wearing their lenses. However, two months later only two of the patients had had their earlier vision restored.

John A. Dyer, M.D., assistant professor of ophthalmology at the University of Minnesota, stated that "Astigmatism caused by contact lenses might last as long as 5 or 6 years."

Another so-called expert was asked the question "If you happen to fall asleep with the lenses on, would anything serious happen?" His reply was "No. Many people will nap with their lenses on. Although people have been known to wear them while sleeping and some even for weeks and months without removal, it is generally recommended that they be removed while sleeping. This is to refresh and rest the eye, not to prevent anything serious from happening."

You will note that he states, "This is to refresh and rest the eye"; so obviously he recognizes the fact that the contacts do not refresh and do not rest the eyes.

The same expert was asked "Do contact lens cause cancer or cataract?" His reply was, "No, there have never been any cases of cancer or cataract reportedly caused by contact lenses." I would suggest that contact lenses have not been used long enough to discover whether or not they

147

cause cataract or cancer.

ARE CONTACT LENSES THE ANSWER
TO POST CATARACT SURGERY?

Frankly, I wish that I could answer an emphatic yes to this question. Unfortunately, from the evidence at my disposal I can't even echo a faint yes. In fact, I have to advise my readers to turn thumbs down on contact lenses, be they for cataract or for any improvement or correction of vision.

In spite of the optical company's statement "contact lens become a part of the eye itself" basically let's face one simple fact ... the contact lens is no better or no worse than a foreign element in the eye. Even the youngest of children have learned the harm, the damage, the pain that a speck of dust in the eye can cause and the whole situation evolves around the fact that the eye is most affected by, and sensitive to foreign objects in its domain. No matter how tiny, no matter how light or fluffy, if it is a foreign object the eye resents it and does everything in its power to remove it. Therefore, how any body of sensible men can justify the placing of a large foreign object in the eye goes beyond my understanding. According to my viewpoint there are only two reasons for the use of contact lenses ... one is that of financial gain and the other is cosmetic purposes. On the basis of the evidence presented to me and what I could learn there can be no other rhyme or reason for contact lenses.

In a recent conversation with a school principal I asked him if he had observed anything concerning the teachers who wore contact lenses. He then informed me that the antics which the wearers of contacts go through in removing and replacing the contact lens is nothing short of a circus or a tragic melodrama. He went on to state that the manoeuvres, the juggling to get the contact lenses out without losing them and then putting them back was an experience that no sane human being would want to go through. He further stated that if it wasn't so terribly tragic it would be hilarious. I've discussed this with other people who have the opportunity to see contact lens wearers remove and replace the contact lenses. Their opinion seems to be similar.

Here is some further interesting information for people who wear contacts and this comes from the top sources.

"Even with contacts you'll still need a pair of eyeglasses for relaxing your eyes and for those increasing frequent days when pollution or dust rules out wearing contacts."

I'm just pointing this out so that you will not be under any misapprehensions about contact lenses. Here these two sources tell us that even if you have contact lenses you still will need a pair of glasses for reading and for those occasions when contact lenses are not readily available.

One well known optometrist referred to contacts as "A boon to the visual welfare of mankind". However, back in 1966 professor Joseph M. Dixon, M.D., who was professor of ophthalmology at the University of Alabama Medical Center claimed that "Everybody who uses contact lenses will suffer eye damage, and in many cases the damage will be permanent." He stated further, "You would be amazed at the number of ophthalmologists who wish contact lenses had never been invented. Our job is to help people see better, and glasses will do that with fewer complications."

He continued, "The trouble with contact lenses is simple: They are foreign bodies — almost always unsterile

— placed in contact with some of the most delicate and sensitive tissues in the body. As a result, they will cause injury, however slight and however remediable, in the eyes of every single one of the 9 million people who wear them."

In his estimate which was based on both laboratory experiments and surveys, three out of every 1000 wearers of contact lenses — 27,000 in all — will suffer permanent damage to their eyes.

It must be admitted that most of the damage that will result from contact lenses is not the fault of the ophthalmologist, the optician or the optometrist. Here are some of the conditions or problems that arise. Some people won't properly clean them or store them correctly. There are those who spit on their lenses prior to inserting them into their eyes. There are those who use their fingernails as well as fingernail files to remove the lens. Then there are those who will make the mistake of putting the lenses which are individually shaped into alternate eyes. Many will get an eye infection and still continue wearing their contacts. Others will go on wearing a scratched or warped lens. And there was the case of one user (there are many) who forgot to remove his contact before going to bed — and this is a documented case — and he lost the sight of an eye.

According to Professor Dixon *"Contact lenses have become the most over sold, over advertised, exaggerated, and exploited prothesis we have. It has even been claimed that they do not touch the eye, which is a lot of hokum. They're called contact lenses, and that's what they are. And every time the eyelid blinks, it squeezes the lens against the cornea."*

A reporter asked Professor Dixon the following question, "If the contact lenses were perfect and had been properly fitted by a qualified practitioner and properly fitted for a healthy patient who used them correctly and properly would they be safe?" Professor Dixon made the following answer, "Make no mistake. Everybody who puts on contact lenses will experience damage. It may be microscopic, but it is damage. There will be minute scratches on the cornea, rupturing of small blood vessels, changes in the cells of the eye, and — most serious — a certain loss of sensitivity of the tissue beneath the lens."

Professor Dixon goes on to cite 10 cases he investigated that involved eyes enucleated (removed) or blinded by contact lenses. In all 10 of these cases bacterial infection was probably at fault. However, according to Professor Dixon the proper wearing of contact lenses on normal eyes would not have prevented these bacterial infections.

Here is the result of a study of the consequences of wearing contact lenses which was supervised by Professor Dixon as published in the American Medical Association Journal, March 14, 1966.

"A survey was made of the country's 8181 ophthalmologists, and 1904 reported on their experiences with 49,954 wearers of contact lenses during 1 year.

"There were 7607 cases reported of eye damage in which the patients recovered without permanent defects. Medication, eyepatches, as well as hospitalization in many cases, were required.

"There were 157 cases of permanent damage by scarring or other injuries.

"There were 14 cases of eyes lost or blinded. All 14 had infections, 10 from bacteria and 4 from fungi."

Professor Dixon stated to the reporter that no one knows what effect contact lenses will have on people who wear them year after year.

"People have been wearing them in large numbers for only some 6 to 8 years. We won't be able to give any long-range evaluation until we can run surveys on a large number of patients who have used them for at least 20 years.

"However, the eyes of rabbits are very like those of humans, and in 1964 we placed contact lenses on 118 rabbits and left them in place for about 2 months. Many of the rabbits developed inflammed and enlarged blood vessels under their corneas. This is a severe injury, severe enough to leave you visionless.

"Many of the rabbits' corneas were scarred so badly that they retained only 20/200 vision — 20/200 is considered legally blind.

"Now, in human beings blood vessels of this kind grow only in eyes that have worn contact lenses for a long time. I have noticed that these enlarged blood vessels appear with greater frequency when people wear the lenses overnight — wearing lenses overnight is in many ways equivalent to wearing them for a number of years. I am presently treating this condition in a young medical student who neglected to remove his lenses for just one night. He had been wearing contact lenses for 2 years with no problems before this occurred.

"But I am beginning to see more and more cases of this sort, even in people who remove the lenses before sleeping. I have a feeling that this may be one of the long-range complications to plague people who wear contact lenses for many years, even if they do remove them at night."

152

Concerning the danger that may result from injury while the contact lens is in place, there is some confusion in this field. One supposed authority (Lawrence Lewison) claims "In answer to a question 'If someone is struck in the eye while wearing a contact lens, would the lens break or damage the eye?' " And his reply is this, "Quite the contrary. There has never been a case of a contact lens broken while being worn — and many cases where it had shielded and protected the eye from serious injury. Unless dropped and crushed, the plastic used in modern day contact lenses is virtually unbreakable."

On the other hand we have this information from the Council of Occupational Health "Contact lenses are not in themselves protective devices and in fact may increase the danger of injury to the eyes."

It is estimated that more than 25% of those who buy contact lenses find them too troublesome or too uncomfortable to wear and a few have been reported who, on account of the contact lenses, lost the sight of an eye.

To deny that there are some cases where the wearing of contact lenses can be of benefit would be unreasonable. I would like to quote the following instance.

"A 23 year old girl had been wearing very thick glasses prescribed for congenital cataract since the age of 8. She was rather unattractive, poorly groomed and definitely had a withdrawn personality. Even with her glasses visual acuity was not better than 20/100, and she had been retarded in her school work and her employment because of poor vision. Needless to say, her social life was nil. Most regrettably, she was resigned to her unhappiness.

"In her case contact lenses were advised. The change was astounding. Her vision, for one thing, improved to 20/25. Her eyes were open to view at last (and they were bright blue and attractive). Within two weeks — when she returned for her check-up, she was wearing a new outfit, her hair was done smartly, and cosmetics were used for the first time. She held her head up and walked erectly. She did not appear to be the same girl at all!" *(1)*

Back in the early 1960's the Federal Trade Commission after being offended by the false advertising claims about contact lenses had a law passed that made it illegal for any advertiser to say that contact lenses:

1. Are suitable and safe for all persons, regardless of their age, health or eye condition;

2. Can be worn satisfactorily and without discomfort by all, or nearly all persons;

3. Can be fitted without any discomfort;

4. Can be worn for any short or long period without discomfort unless the advertisement clearly reveals that practically all persons will experience some discomfort when first wearing them and that in a significant number of cases the discomfort period may be prolonged;

5. Can be worn all day without discomfort by any person except after that person has become fully adjusted thereto and unless such is the fact;

6. Will completely replace eyeglasses in all, or nearly all, cases, or will provide better correction of vision than eyeglasses in all, or nearly all, cases;

7. Which are bifocal are as satisfactory to the wearer as prescription eyeglasses having bifocal lenses;

8. Will correct all defects in vision;

9. Will stay in place under all conditions;

10. Are unbreakable in all circumstances;

11. Can be adequately tried without financial obligation, unless such is the fact;

12. Will protect the eyes unless such representation is limited in application to the portion of the eyes covered by such lenses and does not denote or connote a greater degree of protection to such portion, than is in fact the case;

13. Do not rest upon, or have contact with, the eyes.

From the evidence presented you will have to decide whether or not contact lenses are safe and of value.

REFERENCES

1. Readers Digest, June, 1959, pg. 73, by Mary Perry.

155

12 Nutritional Aspects

It appears as though I'm often apologizing for dragging nutrition into my discussions of health and disease. I want it clearly understood that I'm not trying to bolster my faith in the value of food in health because by actual tests and observations it has been proven over and over again. However, not being armed with tremendous quantities of statistical, scientific or laboratory proof, I am sort of at a disadvantage in many instances when some authority stops me dead in my tracks and says, "I want proof". Now I can give him proof, living proof, of the merits of nutritional aspects in control of disease by my own experience and the actual experience of hundreds if not thousands of others but no, they want it on paper, attested to by researchers and men with medical degrees.

O.K., here is something of recent date. In the August 26, 1971, San Diego Union there was an article and the headline said "Low Fat Best — Diet Affects Eyes Specialists Learn." Then comes the startling revelation in the article. It says "Eye doctors have discovered that what you eat may affect how you see. At the Wills Eye Hospital in

Philadelphia, at Harvard's Retina Center in Cambridge, Mass., and at other institutions specializing in the study and treatment of defective vision they have for the past 15 years become aware of a connection between diet and failing eyesight.

"Dr. Arthur Keeney, who heads the staff at Philadelphia's Wills Eye Hospital states, 'There's no sense damaging your eyes with your mouth. The eye, especially the sensitive area in the middle of the retina known as the macula, is uniquely vulnerable to vascular changes stemming from a high-fat diet.'

"In a recent interview, Dr. Keeney stated 'that placing the patient on a low-fat schedule is one means eye doctors have of controlling a mysterious but common visual defect known as macular degeneration, which deprives the individual of the ability to see straight ahead'.

"Roughly 10 per cent or better of America's sick suffer from eye diseases or conditions affecting the eyes and macular degeneration or involution as the condition is also called is a very common problem in our maturing population. Approximately 50,000 of the nation's estimated 300,000 blind or near blind persons suffer from the ailment. It is interesting to note that this condition may strike all ages, but usually concentrates in the middle-aged population group. The sufferer finds himself 'going blind' in the central area of sight for which the macula is responsible. His peripheral vision is unaffected.

"In most cases a blockage or leak in the tiny blood vessels which interlace the macula deprives the retinal center of its function.

"In treating the disease while the painstaking process of diagnosis proceeds and doctors study the microscopic macula, the patient may be equipped with corrective lenses, and counseled on how to make the best use of his peripheral vision. Once the case is identified in adult cases the ophthalmologist has his choice of treatment methods, depending strictly on the cause. If the blockage in the macula can be traced to a high-fat diet, the diet is adjusted.

"Dr. Keeney is quick to point out that fat isn't the whole answer. It is just one of the areas in which we can do something".

Now you may ask, "What has this to do with cataract or glaucoma?" My investigations clearly reveal that where the nutrition of the eye is maintained no eye problems result but when the nutritional aspects fail due to stress, malnutrition, improper diet or other factors then we begin to have trouble, be it cataract, glaucoma, macular degeneration or involution. I go on record as stating that no one suffers from cataract or glaucoma alone. Other parts of the anatomy must be affected and a close, careful physical check-up will reveal that I speak the truth. Furthermore, I want to stress emphatically that cataract or glaucoma and other eye disorders do not result because you have weak eyes . . . it is because you permit the eyes to become weakened due to improper cell regeneration through the medium of diet.

The selfsame channels that would bring in the proper nourishment would also remove the waste materials. You understand, I'm sure, that all the body structures are sustained by cell regeneration. Every second of your existence cells die and cells are replaced and in the eye the channels that do the feeding and the removing of wastes become impaired and thus we get eye conditions. In this case, cataract.

Therefore, the cataract is not a growth as pointed out earlier. It is just that the lens becomes damaged, crippled and clogged up because of the lack of a supply of the proper nutrients and faulty removal of the wastes. Of course, the medical profession comes along and says we can remove the lens by surgery and substitute a pair of glasses that contain a lens that will give you back your vision. Well, that's fine if that's what you want. I suggest it is more logical and practical to make the necessary dietary adjustments so that the eye can be properly nourished and the wastes removed so that eventually you can regain the use of the lens when the opacity has been diminished or cleared up. I do not suggest that this can be done over night or quickly. It took many years to create the cataract and you must expect it to take at least some months before any great improvement is noted when the nutritional aspects are corrected.

A healthy body requires adequate and proper nutrition. This means a proper balance of vitamins, minerals, protein, carbohydrates, fats and other elements. These must be obtained from fresh vegetables, grains, fruits and nuts. Also, vitamin D from the sun and atmosphere.

Remember, the lens of the eye has no blood supply and therefore the transport of nutriments and the removal of waste products to and from the lens can take place only by an exchange between the lens substance and the aqueous humour. Therefore, the aqueous humour must have a full supply of all the necessary ingredients in order to have a healthy lens.

Now let's here discuss a minute the metabolism of the lens. It is pointed out that there is no definite reason for the lens to require a high rate of metabolism because actually it does very little work. However, energy is required for the maintenance of its transparency for it is upon the transparency of the lens that we depend for proper vision. Also, nourishment for the development and growth of new lens fibers is essential and metabolic interchange is necessary to maintain the elasticity of its capsule.

I will stress most emphatically that cataract, like other diseases, can be easily prevented by following a proper dietary course. Here I would like to quote a series of experiments in which I will give the names of the researchers, the date the experiments were conducted and the journals in which these appeared so that you will have ample documentary proof that nutrition is the chief factor in cataract with the exception of accident or injury.

From the British official medical journal, Lancet, of May 1959 we read of a detailed study where they took two groups of myopic children and they altered the diet of one group by changing 10% of their normal caloric intake by making it consist of animal protein. The second group were not given any advice or change whatsoever. The final results of this very simple experiment were so conclusive that the researchers quickly admitted the influence of protein on myopia. First it should be known that it is generally recorded as a rule that progressive deterioration in eyesight takes place in nearsighted people until they reach the age of 20 or so. Here was a case where the children in this test, all over 12 years of age, showed a definite arresting of such progress when the protein supplement was given. It was discovered that some of the special diet children over 12 years of age not only stopped getting worse but actually their sight improved whereas those children under twelve continued to deteriorate, but at only one-third the rate of those not getting the prescribed protein. And those who took the most protein deteriorated least rapidly.

Among the other findings was that an increase in myopia is greater and commoner in children who refuse to eat animal protein (meat, fish and eggs) than in those who eat it willingly. It was also found that myopic children whose eyes are deteriorating eat less food, yet gain more weight, than normally sighted children. Obviously the myopics have disorders in metabolism which do not allow for the proper use of the food they eat. Could this be due to a lack of food-processing enzymes found in the protein foods they refuse to consume?

Back in 1931 Day, Langston and O'Brien *(1)* learned that 94 percent of their laboratory rats developed cataract in from 60 to 87 days when the rats were put on a riboflavin-deficient diet.

In another experiment at the University of Georgia and University of Georgia Hospital Dr. Sydenstricker reported therapeutic experiments with 47 patients, each of whom had eye disorders. First these disorders were treated with vitamin A and it did not produce any notable effects. Now 18 of these patients had opacities which usually indicate the beginning of the formation of a cataract and six had fully developed cataracts. The whole 47 patients were given 15 milligrams of riboflavin daily and this was the only therapy used. Within 24 hours their common symptoms such as sensitivity to light, itching and burning of the eyelids, faulty vision, and general eye weakness were relieved or entirely eliminated in practically all cases. The remaining cases were relieved within the next 24 hours. After nine months with riboflavin therapy, even the cataract patients became normal in every respect. The cataracts had been reabsorbed and this was considered a phenomenal clinical result.

To prove his point further, Dr. Sydenstricker put a few of the cured cases back on a diet which contained no riboflavin. The same eye symptoms soon returned and again they were corrected by therapeutic riboflavin.

Dr. D. T. Atkinson in an article in the Eye, Ear, Nose And Throat Monthly claims cataract develops because the lens of the eye is undernourished. He reports he has been able to prevent cataracts from developing in 450 patients who showed beginning of cataract by a diet including 8-10 glasses of water, greens such as the tops of garden vegetables, a minimum of a pint of milk, two eggs and vitamins A and C, all daily.

Here let me refer to the paper, "Ocular Disturbances in Riboflavin Deficiency". Dr. Spies and his co-workers (2) treated patients who developed this ocular disease on diets deficient in vitamin B2, with injections of the vitamin. He reported that within 48 hours there was subjective improvement in all cases, with a decrease in the inflammation, dim sight, and ulceration of the eyeball. In some cases, the patients had suffered irreparable eye damage, but pain was relieved in every case and vision improved. Other annoying symptoms may be eye strain, burning sensation of the eyeball, and granular irritation that feels like sand under the eyelids. The eyes water easily and may develop cataract if the deficiency is not corrected.

Here is some vital information.

"Cataracts can be produced in rats by feeding a diet containing 25 to 50 percent xylose, but only weanling rats are affected. Furthermore, the cataracts are only temporary and disappear even though the diet is continued. Human beings apparently are not affected (5)."

Many eye defects are so common they are accepted as normal. According to the famed Dr. William Bates 95% of the glasses used are unnecessary. He claimed that so-called defects can often be corrected by simple relaxation techniques. Correct nutritional habits must be followed. All whole living foods essential to nerve relaxation must be included generously in the diet.

The following is another article of interest.

"C. V. Griffin, the Howey-in-the-Hills grower, has long

163

insisted the reason he has remained virus-free, so to speak, for many years is because he eats grapefruit every day.

"Now he thinks he has found another 'gold fruit' preventive — cataracts.

"Six months ago Griffin visited a Lakeland clinic for a checkup. He was told he had cataracts. When he returned home, Griffin decided another opinion would be apropos.

"A week later he was on an airplane flying to Baltimore to check into Johns Hopkins.

"The diagnosis was the same as the earlier one — cataracts in both eyes.

"Doctors at Johns Hopkins told him they did not want to operate at that time. 'Wait until you can't see to do what you have to do, then come back. But come back in six months for a checkup.' he was told.

"Griff came home again. At the end of six months, which was Monday, he returned to Johns Hopkins for the checkup. But this time he was sure he was going to get a different diagnosis, and he did.

"The doctors were amazed. The left eye cataract was completely gone, and the cataract in the right eye was 75 percent gone. His vision had improved 25 percent, he was 20-20 in the left eye again.

"His doctors called in some other specialists to see what had taken place. The doctors had not prescribed anything for Griffin. So they asked him what he had done.

" 'All I've done that's been different during the past six months,' said Griff via telephone, 'is to increase my daily grapefruit to four. I have two for breakfast and two at night.

" 'I told them that, and they were surprised again. Surprised but delighted,' Griffin added."

The following is a letter from a reader in response to my plea for information on cataract.

"In Sept.-Oct. 1972 Issue of the Provoker you asked for any information anyone had on cataract. So here is my experience.

"When I was 55 years of age two different doctors told me I had cataracts and as I had read in a magazine of a doctor that had arrested cataracts with diet I sent for the diet list, and I have followed it.

"We eat health foods and take all the known vitamins and minerals. We raise what food we can organically and buy the rest from the health stores.

"The cataracts have been gone for years. I am now 70 years of age. I think I average reading three hours daily. I drive a car and average about 20,000 miles a year. — L.V.B"

In an experiment conducted by Dr. P. L. Day *(3)* at Columbia University he produced cataracts in every single rat that was deprived of riboflavin (B2) in what was an otherwise perfect diet. If the B2 deficient diet was continued blindness resulted in every case and once they became blind nothing could correct the condition. However, Dr. Day learned that where adequate amounts of riboflavin were given before the point of no return the cataracts were reabsorbed and the eyes returned to and functioned as normal in each case. Then to prove and double check the experiment, when the same animals were returned to their riboflavin-deficient diet the cataracts came back again.

Now let us take stock of the situation concerning riboflavin and galactose. It is a scientific fact that galactose is an antagonist of vitamin B2 and this can cause a riboflavin deficiency. Writing in the archives of Ophthalmology 65, 181, 1961, Dr. S. Lerman reports that excessive amounts of milk sugar or galactose increase the need for vitamin B2. Now the question we have to ask ourselves is, "Did the galactose in the yogurt fed to the rats create a B2 deficiency and thus cause cataracts?"

In most cases of cataracts there are usually changes accompanied by a wide variety of other manifestations of ill health, such as loss of weight, inactivity and very important the inability to reproduce their young. And remember, however, in the previous experiment the rats showed no such signs or symptoms of any dietary deficiency on a complete yogurt diet. It is known, however, that powdered skim milk has a slightly higher concentration of vitamin B2 than does whole milk. Thus it would appear that the animals were getting some B2 which rather confuses the issue. But here is the crux of the situation. It was found in experiments *(4)* that due to some strange peculiarity cataracts developed more consistently in riboflavin-deficient rats when traces of the vitamin were present than when the ration was completely devoid of riboflavin. Now this is a most important discovery.

I would like to add here that for some years I have made the observation that friends and acquaintances and members of various families that I knew who were heavy consumers of dairy products did have more than normal problems with their eyes, including both glaucoma and cataract. I must further state that in every case the dairy product that was used, whether it was milk, cheese, butter, yogurt or cream, was pasteurized.

It must be remembered that riboflavin is very soluble in alkaline solutions. Riboflavin is stable in a strongly acid solution but is unstable in the presence of alkaline or when exposed to light or irradiation with ultra-violet light which causes irreversible decomposition. The vitamin is therefore usually stored in tubes covered with black paper or in amber colored ampules. While adequate quantities of riboflavin are found in milk I am suggesting that the pasteurization and various other processes tend to destroy, waste or render the riboflavin unassimilable.

It is claimed that the loss of riboflavin in milk in glass containers exposed to sunlight for two hours will run as high as 85 percent. It is known that milk is irradiated in order to increase the amount of vitamin D. Could it be that this irradiation destroys, harms or affects the vitamin B2?

Studies on diets of an extensive nature conducted by Stiebeling and Phipard indicated that the riboflavin content of most diets is relatively poor. If you boil your vegetables and do not use the water a heavy loss of riboflavin will occur. In normal restaurant cooking it is assumed that the loss of riboflavin ranges from 25 to 50 percent. It is claimed that no heavy loss of riboflavin occurs in normal pasteurization. The curing of meat causes some destruction of riboflavin. Also frying, roasting, drying, dehydration, quick freezing, cold storage, canning, smoking, brining and salting. In some of these instances very little loss takes place. In others greater losses occur . . . but in all some destruction of the vitamin does take place.

If you have a riboflavin deficiency you will notice slight changes in the cornea which is usually the first sign. Other manifestations are purplish or magenta tongue and lip lesions in the angles of the mouth. A fine but slightly greasy scaling in the folds of the skin along the nose and ears is another manifestation. Dimness of vision, impairment of visual acuity, photophobia, lacrimation,

167

inability to see in dim light, visual fatigue and corneal vacularization have been described as clinical manifestations of riboflavin deficiency. Researchers have observed that individuals showing poor dark adaptation and a low vitamin A blood level did not improve with vitamin A alone but responded to the administration of both vitamin A and riboflavin.

I want to suggest that the next quotation I'm going to give here might hold the key to the part played by riboflavin in the prevention of cataracts.

"The need for riboflavin in the diet is probably due to the fact that it is an essential constituent of the flavo protein enzyme system, which transports hydrogen from tissue cells to the blood stream, where free oxygen is available from the breakdown of oxyhaemoglobin, and where the oxidation of the hydrogen, received originally from substrate can be accomplished. It is possible that if haemin compounds are not present in a tissue, the oxidation of metabolites is accomplished through the agency of the flavo protein enzymes system."

There is no doubt whatsoever that riboflavin is necessary for the proper utilization of vitamin A.

Riboflavin is widely distributed in plants which synthesize it and also in animal tissues. The best plant sources are the growing parts of leafy vegetables among which I mention broccoli and kale. Dried alfalfa is considered one of the richest sources. Dried beans, brewer's yeast and nuts rank high in riboflavin. Wheat germ is a valuable source. Fruits are not generally a good source of the vitamin. Non-vegetable sources are milk, egg white, fish roe, kidney, meat and poultry muscle. All seeds, grains and legumes contain riboflavin but are not considered rich sources by the experts — but I consider them excellent sources. There is a notable increase in riboflavin when seeds are germinated. In green vegetables the leafy portions and growing parts contain most of the riboflavin. As the leaves get older and dry out, the riboflavin content drops. Tests have revealed that milk from cows fed on fresh young grass contains more riboflavin than that from cows fed on dried or root crops. That is why the riboflavin content of milk is highest during the summer. Fresh raw peas and beans are considered good sources. White bread is a very poor source of riboflavin.

RICHEST VEGETABLE SOURCES OF RIBOFLAVIN

	Micrograms/100 gram
Wheat Germ	480-1,500
Almond	300
Pecan	300
Peanut, Raw	500
Alfalfa	1,500
Bean, dried	Up to 750
Beet, tops	300
Broccoli, stem	450
Kale	400
Lentil, dried	315
Mushrooms	330
Pea, dried	150-300
Spinach	230-400
Soya bean	280-750
Turnip, greens	350

I am totally convinced that in most disorders of the eye — myopia, hypermetropia, presbyopia, astigmatism detached retina, glaucoma or cataract — nutrition is the answer.

REFERENCES

1. Day, P.L., Langston, W.C., and O'Brien, C.S. "Cataract and other Ocular Changes in Vitamin G Deficiency." Am. J. Ophth., 1931, 14, 1005.

2. Spies, T.D., Perry, D.G., Cogswell, R.C., and Prommeyer, W.B., "Ocular Disturbances in Riboflavin Deficiency". Journal of Laboratory and Clinical Medicine, Vol. 30, No. 9, 1945, pp. 751-765.

3. Day, P.L., Darby, W.J., and Cosgrove, K.W. "Arrest of Nutritional Cataract-preventing Factor." J. Nutrit., 1937, 13, 389. Day, P.L., Darby, W.J., and Cosgrove, K.W. "Arrest of Nutritional Cataract by Use of Riboflavin." J. Nutrit., 1938, 15, 83.

4. Baum, H.M., Michaelree, J.F., and Brown, E.D., (Science, 95, 42, 1942.)

5. Van Heyningen, R.: Metabolism of xylose by the lens; calf lens in vitro, Biochem. J. 69:481, 1958.

13 Vitamin Therapy

Please understand I am not a vitamin pusher or peddler. No doubt vitamin tablets have their place in our society, a vital place . . . yet I still tell all who will listen to get their vitamins through whole, proper, unchemicalized, unprocessed foods.

Now to the value of vitamins in the health of your eyes.

When these research experiments refer to vitamins they are not referring to vitamin tablets or vitamin pills . . . they are talking mainly about food factor vitamins. Further, not all researchers come up with the same findings even with similar vitamins but the truth will emerge if you study and observe.

"Vitamin C plays an important part in the nutrition of the ocular tissues. This is established by researchers (1) who found that the interstitial tissue of the stroma of the ciliary processes contains a group of reducing substances, one component of which is vitamin C, which act as a mediating system, facilitating the oxidation-reduction interaction between the stroma cells and the stroma-epithelium barrier. According to these workers vitamin C deficiency in the guinea-pig causes the disappearance of vitamin C from the ocular tissues long before any symptoms of scurvy appear. This loss of vitamin C from the secretory system of the eye results in a decrease in the rate of transfer of the basic dyes from the stroma to the epithelium and in a decrease in the rate of secretion of the intraocular fluid.

"The healthy lens has been shown to be particularly rich in vitamin C, the amount of which is greatly reduced or entirely absent in the lens that has developed cataract (2). According to Bellows patients with cataract also show lower vitamin C levels than do control patients in the same age group and economic status. He has also shown that the onset of the cataract that develops in rats fed on large quantities of galactose can be delayed by the administration of vitamin C. Other workers state that vitamin C has no direct bearing on the aetiology of cataract in animals (3). It is possible that vitamin C is in some way essential for the metabolism of the lens, but there is no convincing clinical evidence that it arrests the progress of cataract in the human eye, although E. M. Josephson (4) believes that the administration of up to 300 mg. of vitamin C a day to patients with cataract causes marked improvement within a week. The same writer states that cataracts caused by poisoning with dinitrophenol respond to treatment with vitamin C. According to J. S. Friedenwald (5) the visual acuity of diabetics, in whom cataract is common, is improved by the administration of vitamin C, although L. B. Owens (6) and his co-workers were unable to confirm this."

There appears to be mounting evidence that while vitamin C is of value in the treatment of cataract and glaucoma the vitamin C should be of organic origin because where the synthetic vitamin C was used the results were poor but where the vitamin C from natural sources was used the improvement was good. Kale was used for vitamin C against synthetic vitamin C.

"There is some doubt whether there is another factor besides vitamin C with an antiscorbutic action in fruit and green vegetables.

"Thus there are clinical cases of scurvy that have not responded to pure vitamin C, but have to orange juice (7). Todhunter et al. (8) report that the antiscorbutic value of a given quantity of lemon juice is greater than that of an equivalent quantity of vitamin C. They consider that lemon juice may contain an additional factor with an antiscorbutic action. Agnew et al. (9) state that a deficiency of vitamin C in guinea-pigs cannot be entirely corrected by administering synthetic vitamin C, but only by feeding fresh cabbage. It is also reported that the vitamin C of raw cabbage and tomato juice may be utilized better than synthetic vitamin C (10). On the other hand there are several studies in human beings and animals showing that the urinary excretion and blood plasma level are practically identical in any one subject or animal when vitamin C is administered either as the synthetic vitamin or in fresh fruit and vegetables (11, 12, 13, 14)."

Catharyn Elwood in her splendid book "Feel Like A Million" tells that the lack of Phenylalanine and Lysine and Tryptophane will cause eyes to become bloodshot and cataracts to form. Vitamin C is concerned with the activity of Phenylalanine in the body. If the quantity of vitamin C is low the Phenylalanine is lost and according to this writer cataracts are created or formed. If phenylalanine, an amino acid, is desired it is found in sesame seed, cotton seed, oats, cheese, eggs and liver.

To stress the importance of vitamin C in the health of

eyes I would like to quote from Adler's Physiology Of The Eye. "Ascorbic Acid — In almost all animals more ascorbic acid is present in the lens than in the aqueous humor, except in the rabbit and quinea pig, in which the lens contains less than the aqueous humor. It was pointed out that the concentration of ascorbic acid in the aqueous is very much higher than that in the circulating blood.

"The amount of ascorbic acid in the lens varies with the age of the animal, being greatest in young animals. More is present in the cortex than in the nucleus *(15)*. The greatest amount has been found in the cortex just under the capsule, and the concentration falls as one gets closer to the nucleus *(16)*.

"What part ascorbic acid plays in the metabolism of the lens is unknown. Since it exists in both oxidized and reduced forms, it may act as a carrier in the transport of hydrogen in tissue respiration. Almost all of the ascorbic acid present in the lens is in the reduced form. Ascorbic acid is necessary for the formation of mucopolysaccharide, and a deficiency leads to abnormal mucopolysaccharide biosynthesis."

Another authority has found through research that cataracts and blindness are caused by a vitamin B2 deficiency (riboflavin).

Dr. C. D. O'Brien and co-workers at the Iowa State University experimented with animals and they were able to produce cataracts to the eye when the diet lacked vitamin B2.

William Brady, M.D., the once famous medical columnist, received a letter from a lady with cataracts relating her experience when she began supplementing her diet with four 5-milligram tablets of riboflavin daily, plus optimal daily rations of calcium and vitamin D.

" 'The last time I had glasses fitted,' she writes, 'my doctor said one of my cataracts was perfectly clear. I am now 80, read all I want to, enjoy movies and television, play a mean game of croquet, cards, etc. . . . I believe God caused me to see your article that saved my sight.' "

I cannot place too much stress on the need of vitamin D in the prevention of cataract. Whether or not the body can utilize vitamin D from synthetic sources I do not know. Nevertheless, calcium cannot be metabolized in the eye if vitamin D is missing. Therefore, let it be known that vitamin D is most important because it affects the calcium metabolism in the eye which is so essential for good eye health.

Dr. Arthur A. Knapp is a New York ophthalmologist. He has been for some years using vitamin D successfully in the treatment of a wide spectrum of eye diseases which include myopia. He has been helping people improve their eyes by this means for more than 30 years. Dr. Knapp is one of the few ophthalmologists who realize the merits of nutrition in correcting eye disorders. In his earliest experiments at Columbia College of Physicians & Surgeons he fed animals diets that were deficient in vitamin D and calcium. These animals developed axial myopia, keratoconus (a conical protrusion of the cornea), cataracts and even arteriosclerosis. These cataracts were similar to the senile type of cataract which is observed so frequently in human beings.

Here is what Dr. Knapp says, "I know of no vitamin which is as important as vitamin D for the eyes. I know of none. I've seen patients take vitamin A, supposedly for night blindness. I've never seen night blindness respond to vitamin A, but it does generally respond with vitamin D. There is a change in thinking among doctors and I think it is generally agreed: vitamin A is not the eye vitamin that gives particular improvement, but D does. I have also found

175

that B is especially useful, or C. It is true that if the patient is deficient in vitamins, as most people apparently are, then by all means give them vitamin A, B, C and D too, of course, for the eyes particularly. Give it to them because whatever improves the body's health naturally will improve the eyes."

Dr. Knapp therefore supports my theory that vitamin D is very, very important in the treatment of eye disorders, especially cataracts.

Vitamin D is readily obtained from fish. Fish oils are highest in vitamin D. However, when the fish oils have been severely abused and mistreated in the processing it is questionable whether or not much of the vitamin D is assimilable by the body. Butter, fat, dripping, cocoa butter, eggs, various kinds of fish all have fair quantities of vitamin D. It appears that vegetables are a rather poor source of vitamin D but mushrooms are quite rich in this essential vitamin. I do not recommend the synthetic vitamin D. I would suggest getting your vitamin D from food or better still, from the sun and atmosphere.

In a symposium, Dr. William Councilman Owens and Ella Uhler Owens of Johns Hopkins University Medical School told the American Public Health Association in New York that Vitamin E is showing promise of checking a disease causing blindness in premature infants. This addition of vitamin E has been administered the first week after birth with very encouraging results.

An Italian researcher, C. Malatesta, tells of the results of his experiments in his laboratory. It is his finding that lack of vitamin E alone causes severe degenerative changes in the retina and the lens of the eye. Detached retina and cataract are two rapidly increasing disorders of our time. It is possible that lack of vitamin E in the normal diet is at least partially responsible. Other research indicates that a deficiency of vitamin E may be a factor in cataract.

From the Yearbook of the U.S. Department of Agriculture we learn "Animals fed on rations very low in vitamin A value show evidence of several successive stages of deficiency, increasing in severity until death ensues. Practically all of these stages of vitamin A deficiency have at one time or another been observed in human beings, also."

For a moment here I'd like to talk to you about the debatable vitamin which was first postulated by Szent Gyorgyi. I'm referring to what was once known as vitamin P. It is still accepted in some circles but is not accepted by the American Medical Association. This questionable vitamin is known to correct capillary fragility and is very useful where blood vessels rupture at the back of the eye. It is claimed to be effective in the treatment of increased capillary permeability. Vitamin P is also referred to frequently as rutin. It is claimed that vitamin P proved to be more effective in the clinical treatment of increased vascular permeability than vitamin C. It is claimed also that vitamin P is closely allied to vitamin C.

Now whether it's debatable or whether the American Medical Association accepts it or not I'm suggesting you should get your regular allotment of vitamin P or rutin. It is found in buckwheat, the whole plant. It is found in fruits and green leaves. The best sources are grapefruit, apricots, black currants, lemon peel as well as oranges, rose hips, cabbage and parsley. It is known that roots and seeds are poor sources of vitamin P.

The reason I'm focusing attention on vitamin P is that it has the ability to strengthen arterial walls. Therefore, it could be most useful in the treatment of eye disorders and in the prevention of cataract.

REFERENCES

1. Friedenwald, J.S., Buschke, W., and Michel, H.O., "Role of Ascorbic Acid in Secretion of Intraocular Fluid." Arch. Ophthal., 1943, 29, 535.

2. Bellows, J., "Biochemistry of Lens: Some Studies on Vitamin C and Lens." Arch. Ophthal., 1936, 16, 58. Von Euler, H., and Martins, C., "Ueber den Gehalt der Augenlinsen an Sulfhydrylverbindungen und an Ascorbinsaure." Ztschr. F. physiol. Chem., 1933, 222, 65.

3. Johnson, S.W., "Cataract and Ascorbic Acid in Guinea-Pig Eye." Biochem. J., 1936, 30, 1430.

4. Josephson, E.M., "Ascorbic Acid in Cataract with special Reference to Dinitrophenol Cataracts." Science, 1935, 82, 222.

5. Friedenwald, J.S., Science, 1939, 90, No. 2337, Supplement, p. 8.

6. Owens, L.B., Wright, J., and Brown, E., "Vitamin C Survey in Diabetes." New Engl. J. Med., 1941, 224, 319. Owens, L.B., Wright, J., and Brown, E., "Vitamin C in the Treatment of Diabetes." Amer. J. Med. Sci., 1941, 201, 636.

7. Elmby, A., and Warburg, E., "The Inadequacy of Synthetic Ascorbic Acid as an Antiscorbutic Agent." Lancet, 1937, ii., 1363.

8. Todhunter, E.N., Robbins, R.C., Ivey, G., and Brewer, W., "A Comparison of the Utilisation by Guinea-Pigs of Equivalent Amounts of Ascorbic Acid in Lemon Juice and in the Crystalline Form." J. Nutrit., 1940, 19, 113.

9. Agnew, S., et all. "Ascorbic Acid in Immunity; Relation of Ascorbic Acid to Guinea-Pig Complement." J. Immunol., 1942, 44, 297.

10. Clayton, M.M., and Borden, R.H., "The Availability for human Nutrition of Vitamin C in Raw Cabbage and home canned Tomato Juice." J. Nutrit., 1943, 25, 349.

11. Todhunter, E.N., and Fatzer, A.S., "A Comparison of the Utilization by College Women of Equivalent Amounts of

Ascorbic Acid in Red Raspberries and in Crystalline Form." J. Nutrit., 1940, 19, 121.

12. Haugartner, J., and Gordonoff, T., "Ueber die Ausscheidung von Vitamin C im Urin nach Einnahme von naturlichem bzw. synthetischem Vitamin C." Ztschr. F. Vitaminforsch., 1942, 12, 226.

13. Payne, W.W., and Topley, E., "Black-currant Puree as a Source of Vitamin C." Lancet, 1941, ii., 596.

14. Hawley, E.E., Stephens, D.J., and Anderson, G., "The Excretion of Vitamin C in Normal Individuals following a comparable quantitative Administration in the form of Orange Juice, Cevitamic Acid by Mouth and Cevitamic Acid Intravenously." J. Nutrit., 1936, 11, 135.

15. Glick D., and Biskind, G.R.: Studies in histochemistry: distribution of vitamin C in the lens of the eye, Arch. Ophthal. 16:990, 1936.

16. Henkes, H.E.: Ueber die Verteilung des Vitamin C in die Linse des Auges, Ophthalmologica 108:11, 1944.

14 Raw Food Treatment

Reports have reached me occasionally through the years about marvelous results that came about by following a raw food diet in the treatment of cataract. Some of the reports were so glowing that I felt as though I could unhesitatingly recommend the raw food diet as a worthwhile means of defeating cataract.

I must here admit that I am frankly prejudiced on the side of a raw food diet. I think it has great benefits and clears up and often cures many or most conditions. Of this I am absolutely convinced. I've seen it with my own eyes, I have witnessed the transformation in literally thousands of cases in the past 15 or so years and what's more, I have testimony from others with more experience than I who claim that it's the greatest and most wonderful cure for disease that exists on this earth. Therefore, I'd be the happiest man in the world if I could say to you and to all who would listen that all you have to do is go on a 100% raw food diet and your cataracts would disappear.

I have in my files letters from a few sources who

claim that they have definitely found complete cure of their cataract by following a strict raw food regimen. However, my closer investigations do not fully substantiate those claims or statements. Now this may be due to various factors. For example, when the cataracts have developed to the stage where they have become completely calcified or opaque, to expect a raw food diet or any other means of treatment or medicine to bring about a complete cure is really expecting too, too much. It takes many years to fully develop cataracts. Therefore no magic, not even the highly beneficial raw food diet can bring about a cure in short order. No doubt, if a raw food diet were continued indefinitely benefits would surely appear.

So for those of you who have cataracts of a very advanced nature to expect miracles from a raw food diet just isn't fair. Now I want you to clearly understand and don't get me wrong . . . I don't say it won't help you and I don't say it won't cure you . . . I'm just saying you're expecting too much too soon in advanced cases. I've had reports of people who said they had followed the raw food diet and the cataracts disappeared but first of all I don't know how advanced the cataracts were and I don't know how long it took for this to occur but frankly I am skeptical.

I positively do believe that if a person with partially developed cataracts would go on a raw food diet along the lines that I advocate, in a matter of months improvement would be apparent and eventually the cataracts would disappear and normal vision would return.

Here is a letter from a reader.

"You wanted some information on cataracts. Mr. Vincent Smudin was a friend of mine, eighty years old, gradually going blind with cataracts. He went to the Boston, Mass., Eye & Ear Infirmary where they suggested an operation in three or four months. Not liking the idea of an operation he asked me if I had any alternatives.

"I sold him a juicing machine and he started in on carrot juice and carrot salads plus vitamins A, B-2 and E.

"We cut out milk products of all kinds and bakery junk and pushed fruit and vegetables more than anything, all fresh, not canned or frozen but not organic.

"When he returned for his examination in four months they were amazed as they couldn't find any sign of cataracts. He died at ninety-one and they had started to come back as he got heavy on sour cream and cottage cheese but this was when he was over ninety and the cure lasted ten years.

"Glaucoma was cured the same way in one Myrtle S. Cameron six years ago and no sign of it returning yet."

The following is a letter from a dear friend of mine.

"About my cataract in right eye — It is improving steadily with my natural way of living. I can see from the side of the eye and Dr. Suominen said it is getting smaller and smaller. I expect it to disappear in time. I really do. It appeared in November of 1963 and the eye doctor told me 'It will have to be operated on when it ripens', whatever that means. I see well from the left eye and don't need glasses. I passed the eye test for my driver's licence two years ago. That's all I can tell you."

Here is a letter I received from another friend.

"I shall be interested in reading what you find about cataracts. I doubt the reliability of the reports you have received of a great improvement of cataracts as a consequence of eating raw foods." — Herbert M. Shelton.

Even at the risk of being repetitious, I say again it has been my experience that practically every condition that is known to exist in man does respond to a raw food diet. However, just nibbling on lettuce or watercress or raw cheese or nuts is not what I would call a raw food diet and of course therein may lie the gist of the whole story. What should be taken is a proper balanced diet consisting of entirely raw foods. This would mean vegetables of all sorts, seeds, nuts and fruits of all kinds and all in the widest possible variety taken in balance. The major proportion of the diet should be vegetables. Secondly, some seeds and nuts regularly and then thirdly, fruit as an adjunct and not as the main course, except on special occasions.

In my own raw food diet I include raw fish and a small amount of milk but if milk is used it definitely must be raw milk, unpasteurized, although I advise elimination of all milk or dairy products in the treatment of cataract.

If you have read the earlier part of the book you will have learned that one of the positive indicated causes of cataract is lack of proper nutrients and poor or incomplete waste removal. In order to properly perform these functions the eye must be supplied with the essential cellular regenerative material in the form of food and the properly balanced raw food diet would provide this adequately.

From my personal experience and careful observations I know that a raw food diet is difficult for all people, extremely difficult for many people and impossible for some people. But I also state that I know no failures where the regimen was strictly followed and adhered to. Don't sell the properly balanced raw food diet short. It is the greatest healing method on the face of the earth.

15 Herbal and Homeopathic Treatments

I have undertaken a rather extensive study of the herbal treatments for cataract. This happened rather by accident. Because of my long interest in plants, being a nurseryman for over 40 years, I came in contact with tens of thousands of different plants and one of the plants that I grew rather extensively in my greenhouse back 30 or more years ago was a plant commonly known as Dusty Miller.

Now let me warn you there are many plants that are called Dusty Miller, in fact, most plants with hairy, silvery, white foliage are referred to as Dusty Miller. The plant I am specifically referring to is properly, botanically known as Senecio cineraria but generally called Cineraria maritima. Please do not ask me to explain the complexities of plant terminology because really there is no valid explanation. However, in the trade and for your needs and purposes it is best referred to as Cineraria maritima.

In any event, it is specifically established that this is the plant and I want to give you a description from the

Royal Horticultural Dictionary.

"It is known as sea ragwort and is a sub shrub with a woody base, the whole plant densely white-wooly, 1 to 2 feet high, leaves deeply pinnately lobed, thick, 2 to 6 inches long, 1 1/2 to 4 inches wide, broadening and with 3 or more blunt lobes at the apex. Flower heads terminal in compound corymbs several inches across; ray-florets about 6 yellow, blooms summer and autumn, native to Southern Europe but has been naturalized in southwest England, Wales, Ireland and even in parts of America."

Now I want to tell you something about my personal experiences with this plant.

Through the years occasionally I came across people who had used the expressed juice of this plant in their eyes as a means of curing cataract. This is what I was told many years ago, long before I had any idea that I would be writing on the subject or even be interested in herbs or in healing. As I was always interested in the various peculiarities or interesting things about plants this was of keen interest to me.

Actually I'm not sure exactly when it was but about 15 years ago I read an article in Time Magazine and I have this article somewhere in my files but my files are so distributed that I don't know where to find it. It told of an American doctor or surgeon who, while travelling in South America deep in the hinterland among the Indians, discovered a tribe of Indians who treated cataract by means of squeezing the juice of a certain plant into their eyes and this qualified medical doctor attested to the fact that the expressed juice of this plant did cure or clear up cataracts.

Of course to me this meant that cataracts were known even among the Indians in South America and that they had somehow found a way and a means of curing or clearing up the cataract without surgery or drugs . . . unless you want to call the dropping of the expressed juice into the eye, using drugs. Anyway, I'm relating the story just as I know it without any desire to influence anyone or to cast reflections upon any other individual or group. Now whether or not this plant that they used in South America was the Cineraria maritima I do not know.

One of the best herbal dictionary-encyclopedias, and one of the most reliable, states, "Cineraria maritima — the sterilized juice of the plant is employed in the treatment of capsular and lenticular cataract of the eye. Its use is recommended before resorting to an operation. It should be applied to the eye by means of a medicine dropper."

You will note that he states sterilized juice and I presume in general treatment the sterilized juice is what is used. But if I had cataract and if I grew two or three of these plants myself, and they are very easy to grow I assure you, I'd be willing to pluck a few stems or leaves and squeeze the juice into my eye just as it comes from the plant. Here I am speaking strictly for myself. The reason I would do it in this manner is because I feel that in the sterilization the enzymes would be destroyed and the effectiveness of the plant juice might be impaired, reduced or destroyed. In other words, I would use it just as the Indians in South America did. Don't go by what I would do but I believe I must express my feelings in this manner.

I have found that few if any herbalists offer or recommend the genuine herbal treatment of Cineraria Maritima . . . why, I cannot explain. However, the homeopathic practitioners have for many years used this herbal method. If you desire the Cineraria treatment it can be obtained through homeopathic channels much easier than through the herbal channels. In fact, there are three or more homeopathic pharmacies in the United States that dispense the Cineraria maritima treatment whereas I know no herbal sources that dispense or provide the treatment.

Here and now I'd like to give you a report of the exact procedure in the use of Cineraria maritima as followed by the homeopathic profession in the United States and perhaps in Canada. Also, let me explain that the word 'succus' means juice.

"Until surgical treatment is decided upon, Cataract can properly be regarded as a medical problem, and its treatment is within the scope of general practice.

"While no conclusive answer to the question 'what causes Cataract?' has been given it is a well supported theory that in general the pathological background of the formation of Cataract appears to be essentially impaired metabolism in the tissues of the anterior eye.

"Therefore, reasonable prospects of checking the progress of the opacity, and prolonging the period of useful vision are offered by treatment, in whatever form, which will serve the purpose of improving the metabolic processes of the tissues involved.

"The preparation known as Succus Cineraria maritima applied locally to the eyes acts as a lymphagogue, increasing circulation in the intraocular tissues, also stimulating collateral circulation and normal metabolism, functions so necessary from the standpoint of the physiology of the eye.

"Clinical observation and experience indicate the definite value of local applications of Succus Cineraria maritima in checking, or even aborting existing opacities. The benefits attained are obviously most satisfactory when treatment is instituted in the early stage of Cataract. In cases of well advanced opacity, and where pathological changes caused by the deterioration of the metabolic functions have occurred, as is characteristic in senility, considerably less favorable results can be expected.

"The use of Succus Cineraria maritima, however, is justified in certain cases well past the incipient stage, particularly when an operation is not contemplated or is contra-indicated. It gives comfort to the patient to know that something potentially beneficial is being done.

"For the purpose of obtaining additional data on the effects of the application of Succus Cineraria maritima in the more advanced stages of cataract, a clinical study by Ophthalmologists was instituted recently in 40 cases, where the average time of onset was over four years. This is admitted to be past the stage when the best results are obtainable.

"It is interesting to note that this investigation revealed that in 22.5 per cent of this group of 40 patients, 13 male and 27 female, average 57.7 years of age, beneficial effects were attained.

"All patients in the series were examined by direct observation, oblique light with the ophthalmoscope, eye chart and extinction meter before treatment was begun, and at three-month intervals for a twelve-month period.

"Succus Cineraria maritima was instilled in the eyes of each patient, two drops morning and night.

"Due to the fact that the cataracts in these cases were well beyond the incipient stage the results attained are particularly noteworthy.

"Succus Cineraria maritima has been extensively prescribed in the treatment of various stages of cataract.

"Clinical experience has shown that the most

satisfactory results are attainable when this local treatment is applied in the early stage of cataract."

PHYSICIANS' REPORTS ON TREATMENT OF CATARACT WITH SUCCUS CINERARIA MARITIMA

"The following reports are similar to the hundreds of reports we have received from physicians and are characteristic of the results attained with Succus Cineraria maritima:

CASE-AGE	CONDITION AT TIME OF TREATMENT WITH SUCCUS CINERARIA MARITIMA	REPORTED RESULTS OF THE TREATMENT
No. 1. Female Age 72	Senile cataract. Steadily progressing loss of sight.	Continuous treatment with SCM for several years improved vision substantially.
No. 2 Female Age 85	Senile cataract. Incipient stage.	SCM has kept the trouble in check. No cure but maintained fairly clear vision.
No. 3 Female	Opacity with considerable impairment of vision.	After 2 years' treatment with SCM opacity not removed to any great extent, but held in check to a remarkable extent.
No. 5 Several Cases	Mostly incipient stage of cataract.	One case with vision 20/200 has improved to 20/40. Retarded progress in other cases.
No. 7 Male	Early stage of cataract.	Considerable improvement of vision; under treatment for 3 years. Vision becomes bad when use of SCM is stopped.

190

No. 10 Female	Incipient cataract.	Continuous treatment with SCM for one year, then at alternate periods. For the past 3 years vision has been satisfactory.
No. 11 Female Age 84	Cataract of both eyes of many years standing.	SCM brought no material improvement, but the patient says she feels better, and thinks she can see somewhat better when using the remedy.
No. 12 Male	Early stage of senile cataract.	SCM after 4 months improved vision — with no further progress of the opacity after several years.
No. 14 Numerous Cases	Essentially in the early stage.	Have prescribed SCM for about 10 years and found its use well worth while. Except in the advanced stages. At times the results in the early stages of cataract have been spectacular.

"The following is a report of recent research on local treatment of artificially-produced cataract in animals.

"In a recent laboratory study, the effect of an extract of Succus Cineraria maritima on the reduction of artificially induced cataract in 79 albino rats was studied, including adequate controls. The investigators produced cataracts in the test animals by four different methods. Alloxan diabetes cataracts, high fat diet cataracts, Napthalene cataracts and 1, 2, 3, 4 Tetrahydrobeta-Naphthol cataracts were produced and the development of the cataract and increase in opacity of the lens was closely followed.

"A spectrophotometric method for determining the opacity of the lens was developed. Seventy-nine animals with cataract were treated with an extract of Succus

Cineraria maritima daily (0.025 ml. instillations) for periods ranging from 3 months to 1 year. During this time the effectiveness of Succus Cineraria maritima in reducing the induced cataract was measured by the increased transmission of light through suspensions of eye homogenates of both treated and untreated cataract rats. Significant differences in transmission values were observed between those animals treated with Succus Cineraria maritima and the untreated animals with cataract.

"This important laboratory work serves to further verify the results obtained in years of clinical experience with Succus Cineraria maritima. Physicians are now recognizing the fact that cataract is often a medical problem and in such cases have found that it is advantageous to institute this local therapy before resorting to surgery.

"Instillate into the eye 1 drop, 4 to 5 times a day. This must be kept up for several months. Most effective." (1)

Here we have a quotation from the Physicians' Desk Reference for Ophthalmology.

SUCCUS CINERARIA MARITIMA

"Actions and Uses: Succus Cineraria Maritima applied locally to the eyes acts as a safe lymphagogue, increasing circulation in the intraocular tissues, also stimulating collateral circulation and normal metabolism, functions so necessary from the standpoint of the physiology of the eye. Clinical observation indicates the definite value of local applications of Succus Cineraria in checking, or even aborting existing opacities. The benefits attained are obviously more satisfactory when treatment is instituted in the early stage of Cataract. In cases of well advanced opacity, and where pathological changes caused by the

192

deterioration of the Metabolic functions have occurred, as is characteristic in senility, less favorable results can be expected.

"The use of Succus Cineraria Maritima, however, is justified in certain cases well past the incipient stage, particularly when an operation is not contemplated or is contraindicated. It gives comfort to the patient to know that something potentially beneficial is being done. Clinical studies of advanced stages of cataract treated with Succus Cineraria Maritima indicated that in 22.5% of these cases beneficial results were obtained. In many of the cases which did not show improvement the process of the opacity was retarded or checked. In certain cases Succus Cineraria Maritima only gives temporary relief or serves to postpone the surgical removal."

OTHER HOMEOPATHIC TREATMENTS

Homeopathic Phosphorus (Materia Medica): Doctor has to determine right dose, according evolution. Potencies 3X to 30X.

Quassia — Picranea Excelsa — Quassia Wood (Homeopathic Materia Medica.) 1X to 3X. Dose: as in Phosphorus — to be determined by the doctor.

Tar-Camphor (homeopathic): (Materia Medica): Dose 3X (dosification by doctor according degree and type of cataract.

Homeopathic Calcarea-Fluor (Materia Medica): Dose 3X to 12X (same as the other homeopathic remedies, doctor shall determinate frequency of the remedy, etc.).

Agaricus Muscarius — Amanita — Toad Stool — Bug Agaric. (Materia Medica). Dr. E. T. Allen, of Chicago, cleared up several cases of cataract with this remedy. Dose

3X to 30X and 200X (dosified by the doctor).

Calcarea sulphuric — Sulphate of Lime (Homeopathic Materia Medica): Has a noticeable influence in diminishing opacities of the lens, partial blindness from cataract; it is worthy of more extensive use. "X and 3X Trituration (Dose by the doctor).

Conium — Poison Hemlock (Homeopathic Materia Medica): Dr. Talbot, of Boston, reported successful treatments with the use of this remedy in cataracts. Dose: 6X to 30X and some times higher. (Dosed by the doctor).

Ferrum Phosphoricum — Phosphate of Iron (Homeopathic Materia Medica): One of the Tissue Remedies. Most useful in acuted cataracts, in the early stages, accompanied by the burning sensation, aggravated by motion, and red, congested, inflamed appearance, without secretion of pus. 3X to 12X (Dosified by doctor).

It appears as though the practice of Homeopathy is fading away and I deem this a genuine loss to mankind. Actually the homeopathic physician was usually a much learned man because first he had to be a medical physician and then study for his degree in Homeopathy. It appears as though organized medicine has driven homeopathy out of the healing profession.

SOME SIMPLE HERBAL TREATMENTS

Here is a letter I received which refers to Eyebright which is a herb that has been long used in the treatment of the eyes. It can be readily purchased from any herbal house.

Dear Sir,

I am a nurse aged 84. Employed in the O.R. Vet.

Hospital, 24th St. at 1st Ave., New York, N.Y.

I went for an eye test for my driving licence and learned I had cataract on both eyes. I was in a position where it would be easy for me to have surgery but I decided to try 'eyebright'.

I made tea (with eyebright) and bathed both eyes and always drank some of the tea. It is a rather slow process. Now I can see without glasses except for reading. I have worn eyeglasses since 1917. — E.F.

The following are some further herbal treatments.

"Dr. Edgar R. Palarea of Guatemala (South America), has successfully treated cataracts in a period of time oscillating between 14 to 28 days (he didn't mention type of cataracts), using an old Indian remedy, known as St. Apollonia in that country."

"The Chippewa Indians (Frances Densmore, 1928, Bur. Amer. Ethnol. Rept. 1927-27, 44:275-397) used, for same purpose the Rosa (Rose botanical name); Rubus Strigosus or Red Raspberry. The Indians used the inner bark of the root.

"These two remedies are used successfully, the first for removing inflammation, and the second for healing the eye. They are prepared in the same way, the second layer of the root being scraped and put in a bit of cloth. This is soaked in warm water and squeezed into the eye, letting some of the liquid run into the eye. This is done three times a day. It was said that these would cure cataracts unless too far advanced. Furthermore, the improvement would be shown quickly if the case could be materially helped."

Here I'd like to quote from a modern book on Herbs.

"Sunflower seeds appear to be a specific for good vision. Sunflower seeds are rich in the essential B vitamins. The oil in the seeds is very rich in vitamins A and D. The seeds are also rich in calcium, phosphorus and iron, all of which are known to be essential for good eye health.

"From an Old English herbal, we learn horehound tea, wine and honey is sure to 'clear the eyesight'.

"Juniper berries are claimed to fortify the sight by strengthening the optic nerve.

"Old herbalists claimed that elecampane 'clears, strengthens and quickens the sight of the eyes wonderfully'.

"One of the great old time herbalists claimed that eyebright 'hath restored sight to them that have been blind a long time before'.

"Rosemary is said to 'clear dim sight'.

"A good drink that will keep the sparkle in your eyes is made as follows: Place one cup of raw carrot juice, one level teaspoonful of rosehips powder, one egg yolk, a little honey, ground sunflower seeds and sesame seeds, one teaspoonful of brewer's yeast, one-quarter cup of eyebright tea, plus a pinch of kelp in the blender, then blend well. It is delicious and an eye-brightner.

"A good eyewash may be made by mixing fennel seed, camomile flowers and eyebright. Steep in boiling water then stain through a cloth to remove all residue. Apply with an eye-cup.

"For pink eye, scrape an ordinary potato and apply to eyes. Also sassafrass pith made into a tea and then applied with an eyedropper. All teas dropped into the eyes must first be strained through a clean cloth to remove any

196

sediment.

"One of the worst things that can happen to you is blindness. Take the very best care of your eyes while you can still see. They come only two to a customer."

REFERENCES

1. Excerpts from "Preliminary Studies on the effect of Succus Cineraria maritima on Experimentally produced Cataracts in the Albino Rat." — Boericke, G.W., M.D., and Foster, Wm.C., Phila., Pa.

16 Miscellaneous Treatments

HONEY IN THE TREATMENT OF CATARACT AND OTHER EYE DISORDERS

In ancient days honey was used in the treatment of inflammation of the eyes and eyelids. The honey referred to was Attic honey which means I assume honey that came from Attica, in Greece, and it had a special reputation as a curative substance for various eye disorders. Honey for the eyes is even mentioned in the Egyptian papyri where it is told that a man begged that they fetch him some honey from Attica which he needed for his eyes. The famed surgeon, Galen, recommended the mixing of 4 parts of honey with one part of gall of the sea-tortoise which, when dropped into the eyes, would improve the sight.

To quote Marcellus, "The honey pure and neat wherein the Bees are dead, let that drop into the eyes; or honey mixed with the ashes of the heads of Bees, makes the eyes very clear." Pliny also credited honey in which bees have died with the faculty of relieving dullness of sight and hearing. In antiquity, honey had a great reputation in producing clearer vision, which may be the reason for its reputation of endowing the power of divination, improving thus not only the physical but also the spiritual sight. Some historians believe that when Jeroboam sent his wife with a cruse of honey to the prophet Ahijah it was meant as a remedy for the prophet's blindness.

The papyrus Ebers recommended that wounds be covered for four days with linen dipped in honey and incense. They believed that cataracts yielded to treatments with honey. Honey dropped into the eyes was supposed to have cured inflammation and other ailments of the eyelids. To quote the amusing report of Vigerius "I have cured a horse stone blind with honey and salt and a little crock of a pot mixed. In less than three daies, it hath eaten off a tough filme and the horse never complained after."

In the July 1937 issue of the American Bee Journal, page 350, a subscriber from New York State writes as follows "I had a horse going blind with a white film over his eye which seemed to hurt. His eye was shut and watered. I dipped white honey into his eye with a feather for several nights. In a day or so the film was gone and the eye looked bright and good." *(A white film over the eye does not sound like cataract to me.)*

Various sources state that honey is still used for trachoma in the form of eye drops.

A friend told me this story.

"A Canadian mother related to him that two of her daughters contracted sore eyes while attending school, where there was an epidemic at the time. They were cured in two or three days by dropping honey into their eyes. It took two and three weeks for the other children in the school to get rid of the same trouble. Cataracts of the eyes were reported to have been cured by the same method, dropping honey into the eyes three times daily."

Here are reports from readers.

"I never had a cataract but my dad cured various horses that he bought for a few dollars due to cataracts and the only thing he used was fresh honey from the comb. If it works on a horse possibly it would work and help a man. The treatment is simple. Just put a teaspoon of fresh honey in the horse's eye, morning, noon and night and usually in 30 days the treatment can be reduced to twice a day and later to once a day and usually 90 days is sufficient to effect a cure."

"Three weeks ago in discussing your ideas about raw foods with out of state tourists the subject of my cataracts came up. I was told the father of one of the tourists had been blinded by cataract. After bathing his eyes in honey for a short period the cataracts cleared up and he now tends to his own fruit trees."

"About cataracts — I would like to report that I had read of using two drops of equal parts of fresh lemon juice, distilled water and pure honey in the eye twice a day. My father had been told that he had cataract so I tried this on his eyes. He was 85 years old and the next time he went to have his eyes examined the eye doctor said there was no cataract. My father passed away at the age of 89."

Here is another method from an old naturopathic treatment.

"Place comb of sage-brush honey, wax included, into the top section of a double boiler; bring to a boil until the wax melts. Then filter through a large flat piece of cotton. Clean the top of the double boiler. (Do not use aluminum.) Replace the filtered honey and bring to a boil. Filter as before, a second time. Repeat again the third time. Then put the honey in a clean container.

"With an eye dropper place a drop of the honey in each corner of each eye three times per day. Supplement this treatment with a good organic source of vitamins A and C. Also, two to three hundred milligrams of niacin per day."

LINSEED TREATMENT

Here I quote a letter which appeared in Nature's Path Magazine, signed I. R. Hicks, Sr.

"Cataract Cure? — Dear Sir: An old fashioned family doctor, who died in 1948 at the ripe old age of about ninety, was still not using eye glasses during his last years . . . He had a great reputation for having healed cataracts, without surgery. I have talked to several people, who had been diagnosed to have cataract operations, and before the operation went to this old doctor for his treatment. The treatment was to drop one drop of linseed oil, purchased from a drug store, in each eye every night before retiring. All of these people had their sight restored — without surgery. None of them are wearing glasses now.

"In recent years there has been great strides in knowledge of the work of unsaturated fatty acids . . . Can it be that this old doctor knew that the growth of cataracts was a deficiency of a type that needed this fat for proper development of good eyes?"

Note: Linseed oil is scientifically considered the finest form of unsaturated fatty acid.

The following is a letter received from a reader.

"I had occasion to become acquainted with a

naturopathic physician in southern California who uses a simple method of treating cataract. She used a particular type of linseed oil which she obtains only from a source in eastern Canada. She mentioned the source but I do not recall the location. This naturopathic physician claims that this method is slow but she uses it consistently in her practice and claims it will give good results".

Here is a letter from a physician from Pretoria, So. Africa.

"I noticed that cataracts in dogs are being successfully treated by drops of linseed oil. I would like to inform you that for many years I have been using, and have been recommending, drops of fresh Cod Liver Oil in diseases of the eye, particularly in cases of conjunctivitis, keratitis and cataracts with great success. Cod Liver Oil also has a healing effect on wounds. In case of infected wounds here in Pretoria, I drop a few drops of Cod Liver Oil on the wound and then dust a small quantity of sulfadiazine powder on it."

From a source in Salt Lake City we quote, "Our dog no longer has cataracts, thanks to an old fashioned veterinarian who used natural methods rather than surgery. He had us purchase linseed oil in a drug store and drop one drop in each eye every night. Today, our dog who was nearly blind, has normal sight."

SEA WATER TREATMENT

A well known eye specialist made an experiment with sea water on his own body. This eye specialist was suffering from a cataract in his left eye. He tried everything but nothing seemed to help the condition and surgical removal was advised by another specialist. However, the eye specialist himself decided to try sea water before resorting to the eye surgery. He tried the sea water treatment for 9 months and at the end of that period the cataract had disappeared.

URINE THERAPY

I'd like to quote one of the most unusual means of treatment that I've ever come across in my whole life. It is known as urine therapy and comes from a book by J. W. Armstrong called "Water Of Life", published in Britain. On page 90 we read "Cataract: before it became legal for laymen to mention the fact that cataract may yield to treatment without operation, I found that in many cases, 10 days urine fast was sufficient to dissolve the film that forms over the eyes." *Again I must mention that according to scientific evidence a film over the eye is not a sign of cataract.* "The longest required was a 28 day fast. Whether it is against the now existing law for any layman to say that he has cured cataract before the law was passed, is a subtle point on which I'm not qualified to pronounce. But in case the disclosure should be illegal we must assume that the cases cured had been falsely diagnosed, since the law implies that no one save a qualified oculist can cure genuine cases, namely with a knife. Nevertheless, it is only veracious to say that cataract is by no means always an isolated condition. What we need to remember is that the eye is part of the body, and therefore in treating the body as a whole for other symptoms, the local condition is apt to cure itself without any direction.

"Glaucoma: This according to orthodox medicine and even to naturopathy, is a very serious condition. Oculists perform an operation, but in many cases the patient sooner or later merely goes blind. In any event, mutilation can never be termed a cure. Patients who have not been tampered with, I have known to respond well on a urine-fast of about a month's duration. As against that, cases which have been surgically interfered with must as a general rule be considered practically hopeless."

Now we should explain that by a urine fast J. W. Armstrong means drinking all of one's own urine. I specify, strange as it may seem, Armstrong claims miraculous cures due to drinking all of your own urine.

The following is an excerpt from a letter I received concerning another form of urine therapy.

"During the conversation he handed me something to read. I had to inform him that the outline of his face was barely visible to me. Got to talking about cataracts and he asked me if I didn't know how to cure them and when I said 'No' he told me. Said to take some of your own urine (unless a person had V.D., kidney disease or etc) and put in your eye or eyes morning and night and not rinse out. He says it's a sure cure and he can show you some of the people that have proven it. Of course the worse they are the longer it takes to get rid of them. The big job is to convince people it's neither a joke nor a trick, then for them to do it faithfully and in secret 'till they have good results to show. Otherwise even your own folks and best friends will ridicule and ostracize you. One woman he knows that was cured is over 80 years 'young' and reads without glasses. So now you have an idea that can help thousands of people and save them a million bucks and also the penalty of wearing heavy glasses."

FOLK REMEDIES

A drop of raw linseed oil in the eye daily. A drop of fresh lemon juice or diluted apple cider vinegar in the eye at night. A drop of filtered sea water two or three times a day. A drop of eucalyptus honey and castor oil in the eye. Before putting any of these things in the eye it would be recommended that they be kept at body temperature or higher so as not to cause a chill.

One drop of castor oil in each eye once a day for nine

days; then rest for 10 days and repeat the treatment.

Here is what a reader has to say.

"Our veterinarian used a drop of castor oil in the eye of our dog recently when the dog showed up with a case of red eye. Another elderly doctor told me that this was one of the best to use for irritations of the eye caused by smog, gas fumes, etc."

OTHER TREATMENTS

Dr. Curtis Wood reports an enlightened medical approach that worked on 450 patients (From his book, "Overfed But Undernourished"). "This doctor's treatment for cataract consisted in having his patients take 8 to 10 glasses of water a day and lots of green vegetables for their vitamin-mineral content, chlorophyll tablets, 1000 mg of vitamin C daily (which Dr. Wood also feels helps prevent detached retina), 200,000 units of vitamin A, one pint of milk and two eggs daily".

From another correspondent.

"As for cataracts my father-in-law knew people who had been cured by gathering ripe burdock burrs and steeping them and taking a small drink several times a day."

A cataract treatment that is being advocated by a respected osteopathic physician is as follows, "If you will take 4 brewers yeast tablets 3 times daily for about 8 months your cataracts should be gone." This doctor charges $15.00 for this treatment. And he claims "During the past two years I have been treating Cataracts with vitamins with results almost 100% successful. The only failure was due to the patient's non-cooperation. It takes about eight months.

"May I tell you about my first patient? A very dear friend of ours who lives in California wrote to us at Christmas time, 1970, saying that she was nearly blind with cataracts. I sent her the tablets to take for the condition. In June, 1971, she wrote that she was seeing again. August 21, 1972, was our 60th wedding anniversary. Our friend wrote to us saying that she could thread a needle and sew, etc. Wasn't that wonderful?"

This same osteopathic doctor guaranteed to refund the money if any patient was not satisfied with the treatment.

Here is another reader's experience.

"Noticing in your September-October number of The Provoker your request for information regarding cataract, or a description of one's experience with it, I am writing to tell you the following:

"As a consulting engineer I am often called upon to do close work that sometimes is a severe strain on my eyes. In the summer of 1954 (18 years ago) I was doing this kind of work and found that in making a drawing, I could not place the sharp point of my pencil exactly where I needed to put it.

"I consulted a leading oculist here who made a thorough investigation and found that I had cataracts in both eyes — in one eye it was quite advanced. He said that nothing could be done at the time but that I should wait until the cataracts had 'ripened' and then have an operation — which, of course would leave me wholly dependent upon glasses in order to see, for the rest of my life.

"This didn't suit me at all. I searched through our local public library and our bookstores here for more information on cataracts. I found a small book entitled 'Better Sight Without Glasses' by Dr. Harry Benjamin, an

Englishman. I bought the book and studied it carefully. It made no sensational promises, but recommended certain daily exercises which it described, to be followed over a period of weeks.

"For the next 18 months I practiced those exercises faithfully. I did them in full nearly every day. Then I went back to the same oculist. After a careful examination he asked me suddenly 'What have you been doing, Mr. Waldo, standing on your head? You have no cataracts in either eye.' I started to tell him what I had been doing but he changed the subject in an off-hand way.

"I have had no cataract in either eye since that time — which should be encouraging to younger persons for I will be 90 years old on my next birthday (1973). I have supplemented my exercises (which I continue to take occasionally) by taking a raw breakfast each morning; In a good-sized bowl I put previously soaked, raw prunes and add half a raw, peeled apple cut up into small chunks. Over this fruit I sprinkle four tablespoonsful of raw wheat germ (which comes in glass, vacuum packed and must be kept in the refrigerator) and add skimmed milk. Along with this combination I take a raw egg and a glass of water.

"This routine along with a disposition not to take life too seriously, keeps me feeling fine and I continue to do my engineering work just as I did 20 or 30 years ago, using glasses only for close work or driving. I enjoy your Provoker Magazine and appreciate your outstanding ability. If you yourself have cataracts I hope you will do as I did with equally satisfying results. — W. G. W."

The exercises mentioned above are given elsewhere in this book.

The following is a letter I received from Ambassador S. Edward Peal about President Tubman of Liberia.

"For three or four years the President suffered from a cataract on one of his eyes and during a medical check-up in Zurich last year the specialists advised an operation. His specialists in Monrovia also confirmed this. Early this year when his plans were being made for travel to London for the operation a lady went to see him and said there was no need for doctors to 'cut his eyes' because she could cure the cataract. He told the lady that he would not allow her to put herbs into his eyes and she said she would only rub the herbs on his neck. She applied the medicine for eight days after which his eyes became clearer and greatly improved. The treatment continued for about fourteen days and when the specialists again examined his eyes they were considerably improved and very little or nothing of the cataract could be seen, hence there was no need for an operation; he only needed to keep the pressure of the eyes under control, they said.

"The President nevertheless made the trip to London and, after a series of carefully conducted examinations, the specialists there also confirmed that an operation was unnecessary.

"President Tubman also had glaucoma and his eyes were generally red and strained but he does not experience this any longer and his eyes now feel stronger and he can see better than ever.

"Moreover, the niece of the President had a cataract on one of her eyes and he sent her to the same lady for treatment; she has just informed him that her eyes are all right.

"The President does not understand how the application of medicine on the neck could affect the eyes but it did happen in his case. The herbs are presently being analyzed and perhaps after this process is completed they might be of some value in the medical field."

209

One man I knew who was afflicted with cataracts of both eyes said to be brought about by stress and tension after the sudden death of his wife, began following the Bates Relaxation system of Sunning and Palming. He started these exercises when the truth about the cause was explained to him. The Bates system worked so well for him that his cataracts were reversed and his vision returned. Except for very light glasses during periods of intensive reading necessitated by his work, he does not need to use glasses. He keeps up with his relaxing eye exercises daily to maintain his improved vision.

One of the eye exercises that was suggested and which I feel is very worthwhile is for all those who wear glasses to try to read without your glasses. Do this for a few minutes every day gradually increasing the time period of reading without glasses. Don't try and do too much the first day but add a minute or two to your reading exercise every single day and start by reading some rather clear or bold type without glasses. Then interchange, read big type and smaller type and in a short time you will notice that you are able to read more and more without your glasses. Then you have a right to expect or hope that in the not too distant future you'll be able to read without your glasses.

Perhaps you can regain your vision and discard those eye crutches.

The following is a letter from Paul Courtright Whyte, an eminent, knowledgable optometrist: "I think of the process as a one way street, where the street condition can be maintained by the traversing individual, prior to actual transit.

"This is why you will hear benefits from all sorts of actions taken in connection with the inevitable disorganization of the eye cells generally or the crystalline lens cells specifically (which cells grow more opaque as they disorganize).

"If one has been experiencing malnutrition . . . use of this or that may accidentally supply same. If one has been toxic, fresh foods, Vit. C will detoxify and help revitalize the gut. If one has not had enough sun on the skin, for the Vit. D reflex (what I call the 'leaf Effect') and the pineal-pituitary response to natural light . . . this can be the cause of the accelerated disorganization.

"Naturally if the disorganization is caught before the cell changes have become structuralized, meaning while still in the functional stage, function can be regained, the process of disorganization slowed back to its normal progression and the individual will retain or even regain cell transparency in the lens. However, if the disorganization has gone on long enough, too bad. What's dead is dead. Then the restoration of sight depends upon surgical procedures.

"I have never seen cataracts disappear in a fully mature man, when they were completely developed, i.e. opaque. Personal testimony must be validated by public verification, in order to be acceptable. Otherwise wishful thinking cannot be discounted.

"I have tested the Dusty Miller product personally. What it does is 'stimulate' the cell function. This means more circulation, more food to the cells, more waste removed. But this presumes the blood/lymph fluid carries proper nutritive elements and that the purification machinery such as kidneys work properly. Otherwise, Dusty Miller use is like waxing your car without having the finish clean.

"The best stuff in the world for telling the eye cells you love them, is the filtered sea water eye wash solution which is produced in California. I use it on all my contact

211

lens patients, personally too. And others have used it on a do-it-yourself basis, for various conditions. Like ptyergium corneal dystrophy, irritation, even to stimulate the brain. The stuff is amazing and so damned simple the U.S. F.D.A. will not O.K. it for national sale unless it is validated by the usual experimental process costing $250,000. And this in spite of the fact that the California company producing it has sold it under a different name than the one I want to use, for at least 35 years.

"If we were smart enough, we could treat the whole body thru the eyes because obviously whatever affects the brain, also has its connection with other parts of the body. This is why natural sunlight has such a beneficial action when it enters the 'unsunglassed or uneyeglassed' eyeball not only producing vision but also stimulating the pituitary and the pineal glands.

"Optometrists who are also iridologists can read the iris (the colored fibers) which is just behind the cornea and tell many things about the body, its strength, weakness, toxicity or freedom from such pollution, healing activity and so on. The iris is a fantastic diagnostic study, so much so that organized medicine entirely overlooks it. But it did the same when Semmelweis suggested that washing the hands was a way surgeons could cut down their role as agents causing childbirth fever. But don't worry about that, everyone can learn to read the iris and understand their own body better, so why pay someone else to do it?"

This is in response to my inquiry to an old reader, a retired chiropractor of many long years experience.

"Home Treatment — In the treatment of the advanced stages of this disease the only hope that can be offered is found in surgery in which case the diseased crystalline lens is removed. However, in the incipient stage I believe that the proper treatment is constitutional upbuilding which will frequently stop the progress of the ailment or bring about a definite and permanent recovery. In the constitutional upbuilding process I would first of all recommend a fast adapted to the strength, vitality and weight of the patient. I would certainly advise that these simple methods be tried in all cases before adopting surgical methods. Give neck treatments, manipulate the tissues around the eyes and restrict food selection.

"How To Manipulate The Neck — Recline on a bed or couch with your left hand extended over the right side of the neck. Use the balls of your fingers and not the tips manipulating with deep pressure back next to the spine. Pull and stretch the muscles. Pull tissues forward and relax forward. Work down deeper as there are four layers of these muscles. About two minutes work will give relaxing effects and then with the right hand extended over the left side give the same treatment of deep pressure. You will find the tissues are sore. This tenderness is caused from congested nerves and as you continue with the treatment the soreness will gradually disappear.

"Neck Exercise No. 1 — Relax the entire body and then turn the head just as far to the right as possible and then turn it back to the left side trying each time to see as far behind you as possible. Repeat this 10 to 15 times or until you experience a tired feeling in the neck.

"Neck Exercise No. 2 — Stand on the floor and roll your head around in one direction 15 times. Then roll your head in the other direction for 15 times. Do this at least 30 times in each direction, then repeat it at least every few hours or at least once a day.

Let it be clearly understood that I give these various unusual, strange means and methods of cures, old wive's tales, folklore, miscellaneous medicines and references for what they are worth to my readers. I want it clearly understood that I do not advocate them, nor do I disavow them. I put them down in black and white for your use or for your entertainment. I will, however, relate that in my lifetime of experience and in observing the various means and methods of healing I find that some of these ridiculous, peculiar, far-fetched means are not a laughing matter because even the strangest of them have at some time or another found a use or a place. I have come across literally hundreds of individuals who have found cures, remedies, unbelieveable results and so-called miracles from the simplest and strangest of methods and means and that is the reason that they have survived and been handed down through the ages.

17 The Sun and Your Eyes

When I was a child I was warned against staring at or looking into the sun. I recall that during an eclipse we were instructed to only look up at the sun through smoked glass. I doubt if most people in a whole lifetime spend a minute or two looking directly into the sun. I have investigated as far as I can the literature dealing with sun gazing and I find that it is something that is rarely practiced by anyone.

However, I have come across testimony from various and numerous individuals who claim to have greatly benefitted by sun gazing and I have reached the conclusion that sun gazing does create benefits, not only to the eye but to the entire body. Now this does not mean getting yourself baked or sunburned or spending most of the day lying in the sun or gazing into the sun. I think sun is something that you can easily get enough of and often too much. However, I am sure that most of us do not allow enough of the sun's rays to enter our eyes.

One health enthusiast with an excellent record in the field suggests that the eye be given a five-minute sun-bath whenever the opportunity exists. Then he claims that short-sighted eyes, inflamed eyes and eyes that suffer from light strain respond most perceptibly to a sun-bath. No one can deny that five minutes is not a very long period and if any benefits can be found by the daily five minute sun-bath I would urge every reader who has trouble with his eyes to follow this procedure.

The recommended means is to keep your eyes closed when you start the practice and let the sun's rays soak into your face and closed eyelids. The motion of turning your head slowly from side to side will permit the rays of the sun to penetrate every part of the closed eyes. It is suggested that this permits the entrance of beneficial rays that can be absorbed through the skin into the body. It is suggested that this aids in bringing in new blood and a supply of lymph to the eyes and the surrounding muscles.

Another authority enlarges on this sun-bath.

"Then, when the eyes are nicely relaxed from the heat of the sun and the motion of the head they may be opened, but only momentarily and when the head is turned to the side. The eyes must not look directly at the sun but may look near it. Make no effort to see and open the eye only in flashes. As this exercise is continued and the eyes become accustomed to the increased light the glance may be directed closer and closer to the sun."

This authority suggests that when this is done regularly on successive days and for a gradually increasing period of time any eye will be strengthened and vision improved. It appears that when the eyes have eventually become accustomed to looking into the sun many benefits will be found by actually gazing directly into the sun and blinking the eyes frequently so that not too much light from the rays of the sun will penetrate so that no harm can be done. It has been established that the eyes thrive on sunlight.

I'd like to quote an interesting paragraph about sunlight.

"Sunlight is very beneficial to the eyes. It both relaxes and stimulates. People who live indoors all the time and do not expose their eyes to sunlight find that their eyes grow gradually weaker. Animals that live in the dark or the semi-dark are almost blind or at least have poor vision compared to those that live in the sunshine. It is a well known fact that mules used in the deep mines in Wales became blind, living underground with only artificial light; while birds, who wake with the sun and go to sleep when the sun is gone, have remarkably keen vision."

This authority stresses that it is necessary to know how to use the sunshine to get the most out of it. Abuse of the sun on the eyes may cause serious damage. If your eyes hurt or ache when you first go out into strong sunlight, for example in changing from the dim light of a theatre to the bright light of the street on a sunny afternoon, this does not mean weak eyes. The pain or the ache or the feeling of strain is due to the contraction of the pupil, the drawing together of the shutter in its attempt to protect the eyes against sudden brilliance. This requires a short period of time, probably two or three minutes before the necessary changes are made by the eyes. All of this is due to the changing size of the pupil, the enlarging of the iris and the functioning of the various muscles.

You will notice that when going from the sun to darkness no ache or pain or strain is felt, even though you cannot see for a period but when coming from the darkness into the sunlight there is actual pain and ache and strain. Therefore, one must learn how to handle the situation by not exposing the eyes immediately to the full sunlight when emerging from a dark location.

217

Personally I have always had good vision. When I was 57 I began to have difficulty reading the smaller print and eventually an optometrist prescribed glasses. I still use glasses for reading but I've never had my glasses strengthened in almost 10 years and I never intend to have them strengthened. Actually I can read quite well without my glasses. The only time I use them is when there is insufficient light or when I must read small print rapidly. I am a very fast reader and I use my weak glasses in order to read more quickly.

Throughout my lifetime when most people at the beach, most of my friends in fact, used sunglasses I refused to use them. Even 50 years ago I recognized that dark glasses created damage rather than giving protection to the eye. I've also opposed the smoked or treated windshields of motor cars that kept out some rays of the sun. I've even learned to drive my car directly into the sunlight with a minimum of interference or trouble. One of the facts to which I credit my good eyesight is the fact that I've never used dark glasses or any other means of protecting my eyes from the sun. I seriously suggest to my readers that you follow the sunning exercise and allow the sun to help your eyes back to health.

Sunglasses are widely recommended by practically all optical people. I'm suggesting that you are overprotecting your eyes with sunglasses and like everything else that is overprotected you weaken and ultimately destroy them. I suggest that if you feel the need for sunglasses to protect your eyes against the sun you are definitely deficient in vitamin A and once this deficiency is corrected by eating foods rich in vitamin A you will no longer need to protect your eyes against the sun. Perhaps wearing sunglasses is justified for cosmetic appearances or perhaps you want to travel or go around incognito. There is no other legitimate reason for wearing sunglasses. Perhaps there might be an exception, maybe you need protection due to some eye injury or for those who have insufficient pigmentation to give them the necessary protection. However, I suggest that insufficient pigmentation is a deficiency condition.

It is related that a German physician Dr. G. Meyer-Schwickerath claimed that his patients with serious eye troubles were greatly helped by the intense light of the sun to which they were exposed in watching an eclipse with the naked eye. Since that event the good doctor has tried to duplicate the power of sunlight for the eyes of his patients in his clinic.

When your eyes get used to the sun you will be most happy at the physical comfort the sun gives to the eyes and the pleasant feeling as well as mental release. It is maintained that the sun gives increased strength of vision and improves the condition of the retinal nerves and the optic nerve. Perhaps the lack or absence of vitamin D is a factor in eye disorders. Well, most certainly the sunning practice can help correct this condition. There should be no lack of vitamin D if the sunning practices and principles are followed.

18 Bates System of Eye Exercises

The Bates system has been the subject of tremendous controversy for approximately half a century. The medical profession has violently opposed the Bates system and yet Bates, the originator of the system was a qualified, licensed practitioner. But he did not go along with the use of drugs and surgery and therefore the medical profession tried to discredit him or have his license revoked. However, in spite of all the pros and cons it is still a fact that his methods helped hundreds of thousands of people and many have given testimony in writing and legally attested that the Bates system does work. The means that he advocated were as follows: sunning, palming, the long swing, the short swing, mental drills, Lexicon card drill and the test chart drill. His intention or purpose was to release tension and stress and to bring about simple relaxation.

Dr. Bates contended that most glasses were prescribed unnecessarily and that if the patients would follow the means and methods that he advocated the eye condition could be corrected and glasses would be unnecessary.

I have in my files many letters, some of which I have quoted, from various people who voluntarily wrote to me. They had no reason to tell anything but the truth and they have found success, help, improvement and cure for their eye conditions by following the Bates system.

One of the attacks leveled against the Bates system was the fact that the book was poorly written, the directions were not given clearly and that there were some errors involved. However, bear in mind that Dr. Bates wrote this book "Better Eyesight Without Glasses" and did this work approximately 50 years ago, with practically everyone in the world opposing him. He did this all by himself without any help. So if he did err in one place or another and if his system was not perfect it is readily understandable because I have read it and proved it to myself. The big fact is that it did work, that it did help hundreds of thousands of people and it is still helping thousands of people.

I do not know whether or not Dr. Bates started the system known as palming. I can find no record of it being done prior to his introduction but since Dr. Bates introduced it, it appears that most treatments of the eye, apart from the medical treatment or surgical treatment, seem to advocate the system of palming.

Dr. Bates insisted that his students or patients, palm frequently. It is suggested that you place yourself in a comfortable position with something or a contraption on which to rest your elbows. Then cover your eyes with the palms of your hands, one hand to each eye. Be sure to cup your hands and do not touch the eyes. Your palms should be on the cheek bones with the fingers resting on the forehead and one hand crossed over the fingers of the other without permitting any light to pass through the hands, so that the hand does not touch the eye itself and without pressure anywhere. Avoid tenseness in the hands or the

222

eyes.

Keep the eyes softly shut. Then when all is completely relaxed, the background of the eye is black. Normally, a period of from two to ten minutes is required for the background of the eye to become black. With some people it takes as much as weeks of practice before a clear perception of absolute black is obtained. Do not force yourself to see black. Do not concentrate on the eyes. In fact, allow your mind to drift away from the eyes. Think of pleasant, peaceful events and eventually the eyes will relax and take care of themselves. They claim that black appears automatically when the eyes and the mind are totally relaxed. Students and followers of palming claim that it is beneficial in all cases of eye strain as a means of resting the eyes in the shortest possible time. They instruct people with cataract to palm a few minutes in every hour.

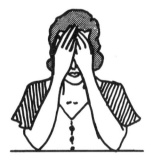

Palming Exercise

I would like to quote an interesting item from Dr. Bates' book that lends credit to the merits of palming.

"Persons who succeed with palming from the beginning are to be congratulated, for they are always relieved very quickly. A very remarkable case of this kind was that of a man nearly seventy years of age with compound hypermetropic astigmatism and presbyopia,

223

complicated by incipient cataract. For more than forty years he had worn glasses to improve his distant vision, and for twenty years he had worn them for reading and desk work. Because of the cloudiness of the lens of his eye he had become unable to see well enough to do his work even with glasses, and the other physicians whom he had consulted had given him no hope of relief except by operation when the cataract was ripe. When he found palming helped him, he asked.

" 'Can I do that too much?' "

" 'No,' he was told. 'Palming is simply a means of resting your eyes, and you cannot rest them too much.'

"A few days later he returned and said:

" 'Doctor, it was tedious, very tedious, but I did it.'

" 'What was tedious?' I asked.

" 'Palming,' he replied. 'I did it continuously for twenty hours.'

" 'But you couldn't have kept it up for twenty hours continuously,' I said incredulously. 'You must have stopped to eat.'

"Then he told me that from four o'clock in the morning until twelve at night he had eaten nothing, only drinking large quantities of water, and had devoted practically all of the time to palming. It must have been tedious, as he said, but it was also worth while. When he looked at the test card, without glasses, he read the bottom line at twenty feet. He also read fine print at six inches and at twenty. The cloudiness of the lens had become much better, and in the center it had entirely disappeared. Two years later there had been no relapse."

224

When I practice this exercise I find no problem whatsoever in reaching the total black stage. If you see spots or flashes of light or other manifestations it is suggested that you keep practicing the palming and make sure you are relaxed and at ease until you see nothing but black.

Dr. Bates also believed that as long as the eye muscles were kept resilient and balanced, the function was performed perfectly and without effort. He contended that eye problems resulted through strain, bad eye habits, chronic exhaustion, general debility, worry and tension.

Dr. Bates also stressed the merit and value of blinking. Explained in the simplest terminology blinking is a quick, light, easy closing and opening of the eye and is done intermittently by every normal eye. The rate of blinking varies with people and also varies with the use an eye is put to. You blink more when you look upon something brilliant or with strong light than you do when you look at something that has soft tones. It is claimed that the dividing point between a normal and an abnormal pair of eyes is the impulse to blink under a given condition. Where the eyes are perfectly normal they will blink automatically. When blinking does not function spontaneously the suppression shows a tendency to become abnormal.

The action of the eyelids in blinking is essential to normal eyes and sight. The fluid that keeps the eyes moist or 'oiled' is produced by a small gland called the lacrimal gland under the outer portion of the upper lid. When one blinks, this fluid is washed down and over the eyeball and keeps the eye moist and well oiled and in good condition. It is claimed that this moisture has various functions such as antiseptic and cleaning action, the ability to reflect light and give brilliance to the eye. The cornea functions smoothly when this fluid is in good supply. The cornea has no blood vessels, thus it requires this fluid to keep it moist.

225

The lacrimal fluid floats out or washes out foreign matter that may get into the eye.

Blinking is claimed to prevent the eye from being affected by cold and wind. Blinking enables the eye to make necessary adjustments to light and darkness or to degrees of light and darkness.

The circulation of the lymphatic fluid around the eye is enhanced by blinking. Furthermore, the eye is strengthened by good circulation of the lymphatic or lacrimal fluid. I suggest it is thus well greased. It must be remembered that blinking does not interrupt continuous vision. Continuous vision is the illusion that a normal eye produces — authentic in effect, but nevertheless an illusion. I compare it to a motion picture which is continuous even though each individual movement is a picture of its own.

It is believed that blinking prevents strain and releases tension. It is maintained that there is not a single instance where blinking interferes with normal vision. It is a natural, essential, constructive performance and improves eye function. However, it is important that you do not confuse winking or spasms of the eyelid or other conditions with normal blinking.

It is claimed that shifting is a beneficial normal habit of the eye. It is suggested that you should constantly shift your point of vision and the reason is that if you do not shift you will stare and staring is one of the worst and commonest forms of eye strain done unconsciously. The frequency with which your eyes shift varies with the various demands upon the eyes, for example, while reading or watching a basketball or baseball game. When reading, the book is stationary and the print does not move, whereas in watching some sport the players are constantly in motion and thus the eyes have to move or shift in order to follow the procedure or the plays.

It is recommended that shifting be as frequent as possible and the normal time required for an image to register on the retina is approximately 1/150th of a second. This allows for great frequency of shifting while no loss or interruption of vision occurs. Make it a habit to shift frequently. If you have good vision gaze at an object, be it the moon or the stars and keep shifting your vision from one point to another on this specific object on which you are gazing. Do this frequently and the object on which you are gazing will stand out much more clearly and appear in its true form as a solid body instead of a flat object.

Shifting is both voluntary and involuntary in character. The voluntary shift is the movement of the eyes by will from one point to another. The involuntary shift is continuous, automatic and very slight. The movement is not visible and is believed to correspond in frequency with the rate of image production in the retina.

When the voluntary shifting is easy and frequent the involuntary is normal but if any strain is produced by the voluntary shift the involuntary shift becomes abnormal also and adds to the eye strain already present.

It is stressed that normal shifting is absolutely necessary for normal sight. Loss of vision is frequently in direct proportion to the loss of motion.

Of all of the exercise for the eyes that I have come across I find one that not only pleases me and gives me good exercise but I consider it probably the best form of general exercise that a more or less sedentary individual can possibly get. This is an exercise that even shut-ins and bed-ridden or crippled people can do with tremendous benefits, not only to the body and to various organs but to the eyes. This exercise is commonly referred to as nose-writing. It is claimed that this form of exercise will release the nervous tension and make all of the muscles and the nerves relaxed and flexible. It is a genuine, very simple form of exercise and all you actually do is write the alphabet or even letters with your nose in the air. You can even write love letters to those you love or you could even try writing business letters but all in the air and with your nose. You'll quickly understand what I mean when I say it is one of the finest forms of exercise that I have ever found or tried.

You can do nose writing with the eyes open, you can also practice this very beneficial form of exercise with the eyes shut. You can do it in the morning and you can do it in the afternoon and you can do it at night and no matter when you do it, it will bring you benefits. You can also do it without being conspicuous even in a crowded room by going through the motions in a more or less imaginary fashion, that is with a minimum of perceptivity. Try it, you'll see that you can do these exercises without actually moving your head perceptibly, yet derive many benefits. Again I say, you can keep the eyes shut, open or softly closed.

THE ACCOMMODATION CONTROVERSY

Helmholtz, using the images of Purkinje*, did not accept that the external muscles of the eye played any part either in accommodation or adjustment of focus of the eye or in the creation of myopia, hypermetropia or astigmatism.

As stated earlier, upon this unproven theory of Helmholtz and Purkinje the entire optical trade and profession stands with billions of dollars to buttress their beliefs. Over 100 million American eyeglass wearers are living proof that it pays to advertise and to put your

* Johannes Evangelista Purkinje (1787-1869). Professor at University of Breslau. In his research in ophthalmology he worked on the functions of the eye and studied subjective visual figures and recurrent images.

money where your faith lies. Yes, most of the 100 million eyeglass wearers are actually crippled visionally by man's lust for dollars.

Dr. Bates' theory was that the eye adapts itself to varying distances, not only by changing the shape of the crystalline lens but by changing the shape of the eyeball itself. In simple words, the eye accommodates itself to varying distances by means of the extrinsic eye muscles with their varying pull on the eyeball.

The eye is operated by six muscles, one on either side, one at the top, one at the bottom and two others passing partly around the meridian of the eyeball, one at the top and another at the bottom. The first four muscles are called the recti muscles and the last two are the oblique muscles.

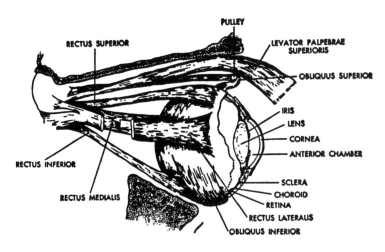

Muscles Of The Eye

During the years of Dr. Bates' experiments which he conducted on animals of many kinds and humans he proved beyond a shadow of doubt that the extrinsic muscles of the eye are the means of accommodation. Therefore, glasses are not only not an aid to the eye but a positive evil, for they do not ever remove the cause but weaken the eye by using a lens that magnifies.

Here is what Peppard has to say.

"When the eye focuses for distant objects, the pull or tension of the four recti muscles is increased and the eyeball is flattened out, shorter from front to back, longer from side to side. On the other hand, if you want to read or look at any near point, the oblique muscles obey that desire by increasing their tension, squeezing the eyeball so that it becomes deeper from front to back and shorter from side to side.

"As long as the muscles are kept resilient and balanced, the function is performed perfectly and without effort." Everything possible should be done to maintain the eyes in this condition.

Now let's hear from Macfadden.

"Clinically and through experiments upon the eyes of fish, rabbits and other animals it has been proven that it is not the lens and ciliary muscle that govern accommodation. The entire eyeball changes to alter the focus and it is the external eye muscles that modify the shape of the eyeball. Accommodation has been observed to continue after the lens has been removed from the eyes of experimental animals or when it has been pushed out of the line of vision. When the external eye muscles known as the obliques remain intact, accommodation will result from electrical stimulation of the eyeball or of the nerves of accommodation. Accommodation is lost when one of these obliques is cut, but will be reestablished when the severed muscle has been sewed together again.

"The same thing happens in the human eye that has been made lensless, as proven by reliable, scientific literature leading back over one hundred years. The usual treatment for cataract of the lens is removal of the lens. The eye then is assisted in accommodation by the addition of glasses, one pair for close work and one for distance, or bifocals — both types of lenses combined in the same frame. But it happens in some of these cases that accommodation for near and distant objects is satisfactory without the glasses. This should be sufficient proof that the lens is not the sole or the chief factor in accommodation, and this fact is set forth from time to time in so-called orthodox literature.

"Either the failure, or loss of acuteness of vision, in middle life, thus appears not to be due entirely to a hardening of the lens. The only other factor of importance in bringing about change of focus is the action of the external eye muscles. Since it has been proven that the lens is not the chief factor of accommodation, the failure of vision at this time of life must be due to some change in these external muscles. This is a conclusion demonstrable by experiment. These muscles practically completely surround the eyeball, and the contraction of certain of them lengthens the eyeball for near-point vision, just as the camera is lengthened for taking pictures of near objects."

It is clear why the optical trade does not accept the Bates theory and why they disregard it and claim that his evidence concerning accommodation is not valid. If they were to accept the Bates and Purkinje theory this would mean that they would have to throw overboard the Helmholtz theory and of course this would mean that the optician business would be sharply curtailed or ended.

Helmholtz holds that the lens is the only means of accommodation. Bates holds that the shape of the eye is altered also to afford accommodation. There is ample

231

proof, in fact, conclusive proof that Bates is right and that the shape of the eye does alter or change to afford proper accommodation but the Helmholtz theory permits the optical trade to stay in business and to thrive so there is no immediate danger of the optical trade and the medical profession accepting the Bates theory.

Furthermore, if the Bates theory was accepted it would mean that by eye exercises practically all eye impairments could be corrected. At no time did Bates stress or use the nutritional factors. If this were done eye problems would cease to exist throughout America and the world. Bates did, however, mention and stress that the general body health was important. Therefore, it must be admitted that he did think of nutrition in this manner.

While I believe that the shape of the lens is a factor in accommodation I must admit there are no positive experiments to prove that the shape of the eye alters in accommodation. Yet it is clearly demonstrated that the eye by the action of the muscles does change its shape. Still, the general concensus of opinion by the eye profession is that accommodation is accomplished by the pupil, various changes in the shape of the lens and also in the curvature and axial thickness and diameter of the lens.

19 Prevention of Cataract

It appears there are two diseases that are more feared by people than any other disease. I used to think that cancer was the most feared of all diseases but from my most recent information it seems that the two most dreaded diseases or conditions are prostate trouble and cataract.

Because women don't have prostate trouble then cataract appears to be the most feared of all diseases because it affects both men and women and, sorry to say, even younger people are now being afflicted with cataract.

There is no doubt about it, cataracts do often lead to blindness and just nobody wants blindness. In fact, there are many who would choose death before blindness and you will see in other parts of this book that suicide ranks very high among people who have had cataract surgery with the resultant partial or complete blindness that often follows. So it is my belief as a result of my studies that cataract is one of the most dreaded diseases that can afflict mankind and strangely this fear of cataracts or ultimate blindness is found in young people of 18, right on up to folks of 80.

Cataract has become very, very commonplace. I dare to suggest that it has now reached plague or epidemic proportions and if you have a father, a mother, a brother, a sister, an uncle, an aunt or some relative or even a neighbour who has had cataracts and you've watched and seen the trouble, the grief, the agony that he or she goes through, then you will understand why people so greatly fear cataract.

One of the first channels of study that I undertook in writing this book was to investigate all of the nutritional factors including vitamins to see what, if any, relationship existed between nutrition and cataract. I came up with some startling but comforting statistics and revelations.

After searching through endless numbers of papers on nutrition and vitamins I found a definite indication that vitamin B2, commonly called riboflavin and once known as vitamin G, was positively involved in cataract. In reading the work of many researchers some of the most conflicting evidence possible came to light. Here were one, two and three researchers who claimed that a deficiency of riboflavin caused cataracts and there were other researchers who conducted other but similar experiments who said that riboflavin had no effect on cataract. Now how can honest researchers in numbers come upon two entirely different conclusions using the same vitamin? This puzzled me greatly but eventually after making investigations and comparisons I came up with what I believe to be the reason.

It appears quite clear that lack of B2 contributes to eye degeneration as well as lowering of general tone and loss of hair. It is clear that vitamin B2 is positively essential for cellular regeneration or as it might be called cell life. B2 definitely prevents skin diseases.

As stated earlier, riboflavin appears to play an important part in the nutrition of the eye. Conjunctivitis and Keratitis occur in animals on riboflavin free diets within 7 to 8 weeks followed by a dullness of the eyeball and finally opacity of the lens (1). These eye lesions are due to defective metabolism in the lens and cornea following lack of the respiratory enzyme flavoprotein.

Evidence for the role of riboflavin deficiency in the production of cataract is most conflicting. Day and other observers (1) have described its occurrence in several species deprived of riboflavin, and its arrest in 89% of the animals treated by the administration of riboflavin in doses of 120 ug twice weekly.

"There are other observations which suggest some relationship between the nutrition of the eye and riboflavin. Dimness of vision, impairment of visual acuity, photophobia, lacrimation, inability to see in a dim light, visual fatigue and corneal vascularization have been described as clinical manifestations of riboflavin deficiency. In 1939 Spies and his co-workers (2) observed in patients suffering from malnutrition an ocular lesion, characterized by bulbar conjunctivitis, lacrimation, burning of the eyes and failing vision, that was cured by administering riboflavin.

"Kimble and Gordon (3) have observed individuals showing poor dark adaptation and a low vitamin A blood level, did not improve with vitamin A alone, but responded to the administration of both vitamin A and riboflavin. This observation may mean that riboflavin plays some part in the visual act; on the other hand it may play a part in absorption and utilization of vitamin A.

'Twilight blindness or reduced visual acuity thus

235

properly called aknephascopia, was considerably relieved by riboflavin, not by vitamin A."

Heiman (4) believes that riboflavin is essential for the visual act and may be a factor in cone vision by functioning in the flavo protein oxidation reduction system and by its power to intensify weak light. He accepts the unproven assumption that riboflavin acts as a photosensitiser in the retina. This, incidently is accepted by many writers as an established fact.

According to Wagner, Richner and Karbacher, (5) riboflavin does not arrest the progress of cataract in the human eye. A deficiency of other factors may cause cataract in the experimental animal, e.g., tryptophane (6). In man it cannot be considered as yet that cataract is a result of ariboflavinosis.

Now we refer to snow blindness. This blindness is attributed to riboflavin deficiency because the diet is poor in riboflavin and the light reflected from the snow, being very strong, causes local destruction of riboflavin in the eye. This is from an experiment from Tisdall (7).

All of the following foods are lacking or completely devoid of vitamin B2 . . . white bread and all bakery products made from refined flour, including foods like macaroni, noodles, spaghetti, pizza, cookies, pies and cakes and also refined cereals. It must be also remembered that pasteurized milk, pasteurized cheese and chemically grown or treated or sprayed vegetables as well as battery eggs all lack or are extremely low in vitamin B2. It is further an established fact that all fruits dried through the means of sulphur dioxide are either void of or lacking in vitamin B2 because the sulphur gas destroys not only riboflavin but also thiamin, niacin and practically all of the B complex vitamins. It is of great importance to note that a high fat diet which is the prevalent diet in America increases the requirements of B2. Be sure to bear this in mind. On the other hand a high protein diet decreases the need of vitamin B2.

Lack of vitamin A causes permanent congenital blindness in calves. Furthermore, abnormalities in both the soft and osseous tissues have been ascribed to lack of a factor found in liver, rather than to a deficiency of vitamin A (8).

Both Cannon and Anderson (9) in their work found conflicting evidence. Their studies did not reveal the same as the studies mentioned above.

We're dealing with vitamin C now. "Vitamin C plays an important part in the nutrition of the ocular tissues according to Friedenwald, Buschke and Michel (10). They state that the interstitial tissue of the stroma of the ciliary processes contains a group of reducing substances, one component of which is vitamin C, which act as a mediating system, facilitating the oxidation-reduction interaction between the stroma cells and the stroma-epithelium barrier. According to these workers vitamin C deficiency in the guinea-pig causes the disappearance of vitamin C from the ocular tissues long before any symptoms of scurvy appear. This loss of vitamin C from the secretory system of the eye results in a decrease in the rate of transfer of the basic dyes from the stroma to the epithelium and in a decrease in the rate of secretion of the intraocular fluid."

One of the reasons given for the necessity of vitamin C is that "the vitamin C has a function in repairing the cement between the cells in all tissues in the body."

"The British Journal of Nutrition describes a study by three British scientists which shows that vitamin C is concentrated in the brain and the lens of the eye, the adrenal glands, the spleen and the aqueous humor of the eye. They put guinea pigs on a diet in which vitamin C was totally lacking and then measured the time it took for the vitamin C stores to disappear from these various parts of the body. They found that, as the animals used up their store of the essential vitamin, it disappeared first from adrenal glands, spleen and aqueous humor. The body retained the vitamin C in the brain and the lens of the eye much longer.

"This suggests that this vitamin is extremely important for the proper function of those two organs. The brain is, of course, the most important part of the nervous system. The lens of the eye is that part on which cataracts form a disorder which is widely prevalent among older folks in our population. In the past, a number of researchers have discovered that large doses of vitamin C will prevent the formation of cataracts in susceptible persons and will slow down or stop completely the growth of cataracts already forming."

Here we have the opinion of an author of another eye book.

"The proper long-term use of ascorbic acid may have a profound effect in reducing the incidence of this condition and preventing blindness."

From the same source we find, "As long ago as 1939, Muhlmann and coworkers, in the Argentine, obtained 90 percent good results in sixty patients with 113 incipient senile cataracts by 2 series of daily injections, for ten days each, of 50 to 100 milligrams of ascorbic acid. He concluded that the treatment had no contraindications, should be tried in all incipient cases, and is more effective the earlier it is used."

Research clearly indicates the importance of adequate supplies of vitamins A, B2, C and D in the prevention of cataract. However, my studies clearly indicate that the health of the eyes and body would best be served if vitamins E and P* were included . . . the vitamin E for eye muscle health, oxygen absorption and co-ordination and the vitamin P to strengthen arterial walls and prevent capillary fragility.

Yes, I fully realize that this is a risky statement, fraught with extreme danger because actually I am laying my reputation right on the line. So I stake everything I own when I state clearly that if your body is adequately nourished in naturally occurring vitamins A, B2, C, D, E and P from food you will never get cataract.

Now please listen to me. This does not mean that you should go out and buy yourself these vitamin tablets or pills and swallow them in bucketfuls. If you do you will not have read the rest of my book and you will be defeating your own purpose so please carry on further.

Here let us get back to our earlier discussion wherein I stated that there was a great deal of contradiction and confusion between researchers who studied the effects of riboflavin or other vitamins on cataracts. The chief reason, as I have discovered, was that they were evidently feeding riboflavin or other vitamins in a pure form. The vitamin was not being tested in all cases as a whole or complete vitamin or complete food. For example, if you use synthetic vitamin C I will definitely not guarantee the results but if you use vitamin C as found in many wholesome foods then my statement stands as made.

In the simplest possible terminology it adds up to this: If you eat wholesome, natural foods that contain the vitamins that I have mentioned there will never be any

* Vitamin P is a controversial vitamin now known as Bioflavinoids or P complex. It was originally extracted from red peppers and lemon juice.

danger that you will have cataracts and therefore I am making it a point to specify natural foods that are the best sources and contain the greatest quantities of these vitamins. So you can protect yourself and your family from ever having cataract by the ingestion or the frequent serving of these foods on your table.

At the same time I want to make it crystal clear that if you feed these foods containing these vitamins to your family not only will they not contract cataract but the chances are they'll have few, if any, other diseases.

In my opinion, based on my studies, here is how to prevent cataracts from ever happening to your eyes. Without any doubt whatsoever a properly balanced diet in itself would be sufficient to prevent cataracts. However, just what constitutes a proper or perfect diet is a matter of great conjecture. Because I have spent more than fifteen years intensively studying nutrition and diet I feel I can 'guess' as closely as any living man.

So you say you are ready to listen to me and you are waiting for the diet that I advise to rid yourself of cataracts or to prevent cataracts and glaucoma.

We start with a big raw salad at least once a day but preferably twice a day. Each salad must contain a minimum of 8 to 10 different vegetables and I'm listing them so that this will not be left to chance. Remember, these are to be eaten uncooked and fresh. Here is the list from which you can select:

lettuce	radish	spinach	escarole
celery	parsley	watercress	asparagus
cucumber	cabbage	beans, green	onion
tomato	peas, green	kale	beet
pepper	carrot	endive	broccoli
cauliflower	turnip	garlic	

Use no commercial dressing whatsoever ... use a mixture of cider vinegar and oil or raw egg.

Then once a day you should have a serving of raw cereal. The cereal must be eaten entirely raw. Here is the formula for the cereal.

Without boasting it is the finest, the best balanced, the most nutritious assembled food in the whole world.

Whole Oats	10 parts
Whole Barley	2 parts
Whole Wheat	2 parts
Whole Rye	2 parts
Whole Buckwheat	2 parts
Whole Millet	2 parts
Whole Sesame	1 part
Flax	1 part
Alfalfa Herb, Powdered	2 parts
Dried Prunes	2 parts
Dried Raisins	2 parts
Dried Peaches	1 part
Dried Apricots	2 parts
Dried Dates	1 part
Dried Figs	1 part

Total — 15 Ingredients

Cut fruits into small pieces. Thoroughly mix fruits and grains together.

Don't cook or heat ... just add water — spring or well water preferred ... let soak overnight.

Add milk, cold or warm (never hot), if desired. Eat 2 to 3 heaping teaspoons every day or at least every other day. Usually I add a fresh sliced banana or fruits in season. This makes it a perfect food from a nutritional viewpoint. You will also find that when you have adjusted to the cereal that it is also the perfect food for taste.

I make a batch to last about a week and keep it in the refrigerator.

Maybe fifteen ingredients are not essential at one time. But remember, I am trying to help busy people keep healthy by means of proper, natural, uncooked, untreated food in this modern day, and this way is safe and sure.

Make certain that none of these grains or fruits have been heated, steamed, sulphured or otherwise chemically treated.

For people with dentures it may be adviseable to grind the seeds before mixing with the fruits. Whenever I have a guest who has dentures I always have a bag of the mixed seeds on hand and grind the required amount at the table. It takes but 10 seconds by actual timing in a small electric grinder. Then I simply add some cut dates, a sliced banana and a dash of milk and my dentured friend is perfectly nourished.

Besides this you have a choice of various kinds of nuts but the nuts must be fresh out of the shell. You cannot buy them shelled because this means the nutrient value has been lost or impaired. This diet will definitely show improvement in every instance.

The above foods contain adequate quantities of vitamins A, B, C, E, K and P. Then add some vitamin D from the sun and atmosphere and you have complete protection against cataract.

REFERENCES

1. Day, P.L., Langston, W.C., and O'Brien, C.S. "Cataract and other Ocular Changes in Vitamin G Deficiency." Am. J. Ophth., 1931, 14, 1005; O'Brien, C.S. "Experimental Cataract in Vitamin G. Deficiency." Arch. Ophth., 1932, 8, 880; Day, P.L., and Langston, W.C. "Further Experiments with Cataract in Albino Rats resulting from the Withdrawal of Vitamin G from the Diet." J. Nutrit., 1934, 7. 97; Day, P.L., Darby, W.J., and Cosgrove, K.W. "Arrest of Nutritional Cataract-preventing Factor." J. Nutrit., 1937, 13, 389.

2. Spies, T., Vilter, R.W., and Asche, W.F. "Pellagra, Beriberi and Riboflavin Deficiency in Human Beings." J. Amer. Med. Ass., 1939, 113, 931; Spies, T.D., Bean, W.B., and Ashe, W.F. "Recent Advances in the Treatment of Pellagra and Associated Deficiencies." Ann. Int. Med., 1939, 12, 1830.

3. Kimble, M.S., and Gordon, E.S. "The Importance of Riboflavin and Ascorbic Acid in the Utilization of Vitamin A". J. Biol. Chem., 1939, 128, 1ii.

4. Heiman, M. "Riboflavin: Significance of its Photodynamic Action and importance of its Properties for the Visual Act." Arch. Ophthal., 1942, 28, 492.

5. Wagner, H., Richner, H., and Karbacher, P. "Vorlaufiges Ergebnis der Therapie des Altersstars mit Vitamin B2 (Lactoflavin) — Verabreichung; Kontrolle mit Spaltlampenmikroskopie." Klin. Monatsbl. f. Augenh., Oct., 1938, 101, 537-543.

6. Albanese, A.A., and Buschke, W. "On Cataract and Certain Other Manifestations of Tryptophane Deficiency in Rats." Science, 1942, 95, 584.

7. Tisdall, F.F., McCreary, J.F., and Pearce, H. "The Effect of Riboflavin on Corneal Vascularization and Symptoms of Eye Fatigue in R.C.A.F. Personnel." Canad. Med. Ass. J., 1943, 49, 5.

8. Hart, G.H. "Vitamin A Deficiency and Requirements of Farm Mammals." Nutrit. Abs. Rev., 1940, 10, 10.; Warkany, J., and Nelson, R.C. "Congenital Deformities occurring in the Offspring of Rats reared on deficient Diets." J. Nutrit., 1942, 23, 321.

9. Cannon, M.D. "Failure of Maternal Vitamin A Depletion to produce congenital Abnormalities in the Young of Rats." Proc. Soc. Exp. Biol. Med., 1940, 44, 44, 129.; Anderson, D.H. "Incidence of congenital diaphragmatic Hernia in the Young of Rats bred on a Diet deficient in Vitamin A." Am. J. Dis. Child., 1941, 62, 888.

10. Friedenwald, J.S., Buschke, W., and Michel, H.O. "Role of Ascorbic Acid in Secretion of Intraocular Fluid." Arch. Ophthal., 1943, 29, 535.

20 I Have Cataracts—I Don't Want Surgery. What Can I Do?

In writing this book on cataract I have done as I always do when writing a book . . . I devote myself body and soul, heart, mind, spirit, and whatever other faculties I possess or can borrow to studying my subject thoroughly. I go to great ends to get information. I actually go to every source no matter how ridiculous, how unusual, how strange.

From my discussions and investigations on the eyes one conclusion I have reached is that when cataracts have been allowed to develop to the stage where there is complete opacity there appears to be no other avenue left but surgery. I have actually seen such cases among older people. I've also seen such cases where the doctor has recommended that the patient wait until the cataracts were 'ripe' as the doctors call it.

I have no intention of fighting a pitched battle with the medical profession or with medical concensus of opinion but I believe — and have seen more than ample proof — that cataracts can in most cases be cured without

245

surgery or drugs. However, I have never known or read of any cases of fully developed cataracts being cured or helped by any other means except surgery. By this I'm suggesting that when the cataract has been allowed to progress to the stage where complete degeneration has set in . . . to expect to turn the clock back is actually expecting a miracle and it would take a miracle to bring back vision under such circumstances.

Actually, I have received reports from hundreds of people through the years that claim clearly and decisively that if the cataracts have not developed too far, their progress can positively be arrested and stopped right there, immediately by following various natural procedures. Then slowly but surely the condition can be improved until vision gets back to normal but this depends to a great extent upon the effort that the individual is willing to make.

Various methods are given in this book. Some even border on the ridiculous but then most or many people think that spiritual healing is ridiculous. There is no quarrelling with results and no matter what method was pursued and followed as long as it brought results or cures then who am I to say that it should not be done or that it's ridiculous?

When the first signs or the early stages of cataract have begun and you become aware of this and you go to a doctor and he diagnoses your condition as being cataract there is still ample time to use the various natural treatments to relieve or correct the condition so that surgery will not be necessary. *This is an emphatic, positive, true, scientifically established statement, no matter what the AMA or anyone else says to the contrary.*

It appears to be clear that two important causative factors are involved in cataracts. First and by far the most

246

important is the nutritional aspect and the second is the stress or tension factor. I do feel that nutrition is by far the most important. Many established authorities feel and clearly state that tension and stress are the prime contributors to cataract. In view of this strong stand I am rather loathe to take a firm or positive stand on nutrition. However, I must do as my studies and conscience dictate.

So if we want to prevent cataracts or if we want to treat them successfully without surgery or drugs then we have to combine the treatment — relieve the stress and the pressure and make sure that the body is adequately nourished, especially with such foods as will help correct the existing condition.

From those who have used the various methods that I advocate I learned that by correcting the nutritional aspects and removing the stress the progress of the cataract can be positively stopped within a very short time and from there on the condition should improve until normal or close to normal vision has returned.

You will recall that earlier I mentioned that stress causes a stricture which prevents the nutrients from being carried to the lens and also impedes the removal of the wastes. So we release the stress by resolve or capable instructions and help. Thus the channels are cleared and now with proper nutrition the lens can be fed and nourished and, equally important, at the same time the waste matter can be removed. The end result is that the cloudiness and the grayness fade away and normal vision is returned. The precise manner in which this works has yet not been completely explained or understood but we do know there are constructive and destructive changes constantly going on in the lens as well as in every other living cell. One. authority claims that "senile cataract is usually a local manifestation of the entire body, a nutrition, electrochemical imbalance."

I must go on record as stating that I do not believe it is always advisable to treat one's self but I do not for a moment suggest that this cannot be done. I would have no fear or qualms whatsoever in treating myself as I have done with most of the problems that have arisen throughout my lifetime. I also admit that there were occasions where I sought medical, chiropractic and naturopathic advice. However, with the knowledge that I have gained, today I believe that I could manage very well and would require no advice from any other source.

If I were put in a predicament where someone said to me "Now let's be candid, now let's get to the point. If you discovered that you had cataract and it was scientifically established that it was cataract what would you do?" I would have to reply in this manner.

In the first place, knowing my diet and my way of life I don't think it is possible for me to get senile or degenerative cataract. But assuming that I lived conventionally and my condition was diagnosed as the beginning of cataract and knowing what I know today, that is with my present fund of nutritional and biological knowledge, I would immediately go on a chiefly raw food diet. I would try to make it 100% raw but realizing perfection is difficult to attain I would be content with a mainly raw food diet.

Then realizing the importance of the scientifically proven fact that vitamins A, B2, C, D and E are absolutely essential I would make sure that my diet included ample quantities of foods that are loaded with these vitamins. Then I would eliminate all possible degenerating influences such as liquor, tobacco, coffee and others. I would eliminate all animal fats from the diet, eliminate all dairy products from the diet, eliminate sugar in any form, white, brown, yellow or any other kind of sugar. Now this does not mean the exclusion of unpasteurized honey or fruits, fresh or dried.

Exposure to sunlight of the head, face, eyes, hands and to the body must be provided even during the winter months. Remember, vitamin D in its best form from the sun, is absolutely essential for proper metabolization of vitamin C. Vitamins as found only in natural food permit the functioning and metabolization of all the vitamins.

I would avoid all foods or substances that may contain mineral oil, take no drug laxatives of any kind. Remember that mineral oils are applied to many products including such vegetables as cucumbers, green peppers, turnips, apples, dehydrated fruits, dehydrated vegetables, egg white solids and there may be others. Remember also, vitamin A is necessary to loosen or diffuse calcium. Therefore, to cause the cataract to be reabsorbed a vitamin A-calcium balance must be maintained.

I feel certain that by following this line of treatment I would correct the condition in a comparatively short time but even then I would not change from my new way of living because if it brought about a cure or a correction of a condition then I would know I was on the right track and I would never deviate again.

Furthermore, I would include in my regimen the basic principles taught by Dr. Bates which are widely known as the sunning, swinging and palming exercises. Now the reason that I would add this therapy is that I feel that these exercises can't possibly do any harm and from studies, case histories and personal discussions no doubt they could do a great deal of good. In other words, I would want to aid my eyes and my body to correct the eye condition in the best possible manner and I would do nothing that could possibly harm that process. Since I began making my investigations on the cataract study I have made it a point to keep in touch with people who were trying or following these various means and methods of cure and I will cite specifically that some were using the Cineraria maritima method, some were using the concentrated food supplements, some were using the 100% raw food diet method and each definitely reported improvement and some that the cataracts had not developed any further. In none of the cases did I receive word that there was no positive benefit.

There is no doubt in my mind that in some cases there would be no improvement even though I did not receive that news. The reason that I say there must be some cases where there was no improvement is because not every one of us has the ability or the stamina to follow through on these treatments or these means of cure because they are difficult in many instances. Therefore, some must fall by the wayside and the treatment fail but in honesty I state that none reported back to me that the treatment did not bring improvement.

So the obvious conclusion that I've reached is that those who had improvement took the time and trouble to notify me whereas those who did not have improvement just ignored my request for further information. This is my opinion, I have no proof of this, but after bearing down on the subject for approximately 10 years and not hearing any adverse reactions or failures I am led to the positive conclusion that these natural methods do work and bring results and no one can deny that I have placed the entire situation before you without any attempt to hide or cover up anything.

It is my belief that the basic cause of cataract is the contraction of the channels that supply the lens with nutrients and remove the wastes. When this condition by various means is corrected and the essential nutrition is supplied to the lens and the waste removed, the condition improves or completely clears up, thus no cataract.

Supplying nutrition and removing wastes is a perfect circle.
Be good to your eyes and your eyes will be good to you.

21 Why America is Becoming Blind

There is an excellent publication called "I Didn't See It" put out by the American Optometric Association. It is well written, well prepared and in many ways makes good sense.

I want to quote you a few pages from this small booklet and this particular section is entitled "How To Improve Your Vision".

"Thorough Analysis — Basic to any correction by a vision specialist is a thorough visual analysis to determine what, if any, inefficiencies you have. The old-fashioned test of reading letters on a chart twenty feet away is inadequate. That is a test for distance acuity only. It reveals nothing about depth perception, field of vision, night blindness, or co-ordination — the ability of the two eyes to work together. All of these are important to safe driving. Modern optometric analysis covers all.

"Lenses — Unless your lenses are prescribed to take into account all the important facts found in a complete analysis, they will not correct your vision, and they may unnecessarily handicap one skill while correcting another. That is why you need the services of a vision specialist who gives you a thorough visual analysis from the standpoint of everyday needs. He will consider individual requirements in driving, whether you drive a truck for a living, or a pleasure car just over week-ends; whether you do much night driving; whether most of your driving is in heavy city traffic where your problems are close at hand, or on fast highways where more distant vision is important. Your vision specialist will prescribe as he deems necessary in the form of lenses or training to insure proper corrective measures to fit the requirements of the case.

"Visual training, or orthoptics, is a relatively new form of correction. In nontechnical terms it consists of "eye exercises" — correction of faulty visual habits, and development of necessary visual skills. This form of training to re-educate and train visual perception came into prominence during the war, when it was used extensively to train aviators. It is used in the offices of many vision specialists to improve visual co-ordination and efficiency.

"Seeing is not a simple mechanical process, like a camera recording a picture on a film. We must have healthy eyes to see, but good vision takes more than that. Good vision requires co-ordination of many muscles and nerves, and it is a learned skill. As children, we learn to see just as we learn to crawl, walk, and talk. In that learning, we sometimes fail to develop the proper visual skills, therefore visual training is frequently necessary to correct seeing problems. It may be prescribed in conjunction with lenses, or without them, as an aid to proper adaptation of seeing skills to the adequate performance of everyday tasks. Visual training can often make it possible for drivers to meet qualifications for driving licenses, because, by visual training, the motorist learns to see faster and more widely. Therefore it is a type of correction that every driver should know about. Adequate and efficient vision is a vital factor in making driving safer, and to acquire such vision drivers should take advantage of the most advanced methods known to science."

I must agree in total with most of the statements made and their aim but I have some very nasty questions to ask. How come the aborigenes and animals have good or perfect vision without all the gimmicks suggested by this pamphlet?

I note that nowhere is nutrition mentioned. Now I know for certain that the Optometic Association have one thing to sell and that is their services and glasses and from all the literature that I've read their chief interest and aim in life is to sell these glasses. It is my contention that glasses never correct anything. They do not make your eyes stronger, they make them weaker. They may enable you to read but the same glasses will not let you see at any great distance, at least not well. They do not mention that at best glasses are only crutches and that they really correct nothing. However, through long years of nutritional studies I know that eye conditions can be corrected and the eyes brought back into functional use by means of nutrition and perhaps eye exercises. You see there is no money in nutrition and there is no money in eye exercises but there is lots of money in selling glasses. I trust you get the point.

Here we have the views of the Better Vision Institute.

"By urging all Americans to have regular eye examinations and to take care of their eyes, the Better Vision Institute (BVI) brings patients to the eye doctor, customers to the optician, and increases the market for supply houses and manufacturers.

"How does BVI tell the story of good eye care? BVI uses television, radio, magazines, newspapers, movies, plant

255

posters — all media — to reach millions of Americans each year. Because BVI is a non-profit, educational organization providing useful, accurate information, its material is well received — and widely used — by the press. Television stations broadcast — and rebroadcast — BVI one-minute announcements on eye care. Radio stations receive recorded announcements and special features."

I wonder if the BVI is not more interested in making money for the eye practitioners and the optical companies than it is in providing good vision for the American people.

I have a publication called Vision Literature Catalogue, published by the American Optometric Association. It is a well printed, 20 page booklet with an interesting cover and contains the best of literature and advertising material for the eyes, or should I say for the benefit of the eye practitioners. These are mainly for practitioners to buy and distribute to their clientele or through the mail. It is an exceptionally fine catalogue and must do a tremendous job in promoting the use of eye glasses and contact lens. From all of this I can plainly see that there is a tremendous selling campaign coupled with aid from the best Madison Avenue writers and advertising specialists, paid for by the people in the optical trade to sell crutches instead of ways and means to avoid ruining or destroying the eyes. If the government would conduct a campaign to teach people, young and old, to eat right there would be no need for these eye crutches or even for most healers.

I am greatly impressed by the tremendous flood of literature distributed by the optical practitioners and trade. I think they do even a better job than the American Medical Association. I gather further that the optical lens trade or business is very tightly controlled. Their literature is very well written and planned with one aim, to make us believe that the optical trade and practitioners are angels

256

sent by heaven to correct the errors of nature in making poor eyes. As I see it, it is the aim of the medical profession through the ophthalmologists as well as the opticians and optometrists to make us dependent upon eye crutches which they supply at high to fancy prices.

I am not suggesting that the optical trade and profession prescribe glasses for children and adults with perfect vision or that they are cheating anyone or are responsible for the poor eyesight of the nation. I emphasize, I make no such accusation nor have I any reason or justification for so suggesting. However, I do specify clearly with all the strength at my command that if the optical trade and profession really wanted to help the children and adults they would investigate and learn that I speak the truth when I state that 95% or better of all reasons for prescribing and fitting glasses could be eliminated if proper nutrition and eye exercises were practiced.

I would further state that the optical profession and trade is no worse in any manner, shape or form than the medical profession or the drug manufacturers. My big, big gripe is that children are crippled for life by the entire optical trade when they slap glasses practically on infants and from that moment on they become dependent upon these crutches and their eyes grow progressively weaker. Naturally the parents are basically to blame. However, the government should be honest enough and big enough to direct the parents to proper nutrition but as the government is controlled by various vested interests such as the optical and drug industries no help can be expected from government sources and thus the eyes of infants and children will continue to be sacrificed so that the optical trade and profession can grow wealthy.

The following was quoted from information furnished by the Better Vision Institute.

257

"It is estimated that one out of two Americans, or about 100 million people wear eyeglasses today. By 1975, it is estimated that two out of three Americans will be wearing eyeglasses.

"It is estimated that ten million Americans have purchased contact lenses, but the number of actual wearers is unknown. Each year, about 600 thousand people (3/5 of a million) are fitted with contact lenses."

"Progress In A Nutshell — The number of people five years and older who wear eyeglasses has increased by about one-third . . . from 76 million in 1956 to 99 million in 1966. The gain is 23 million people. Two-fifths of this gain (9 million) may be attributed to factors other than population growth. (In 1968, the Better Vision Institute estimates that this 99 million figure has increased to 100 million).

"The greatest inroads have been made among young people age five to nineteen.

"In 1956 there were some 8 million youngsters in this age group who wore eyeglasses. Now, there are 17 million. In other words, the number of eyeglass wearers in this age group has better than doubled during the past ten years. The gain is 9 million youngsters. Two-thirds of this (6 million) may be attributed to factors other than growth of this age group.

"A Profile Of The Eyeglass Wearer — 1966 vs. 1956. — While the total population 5 years and older has increased by about one-fifth since 1956, the number of people wearing eyeglasses in this age group has increased by nearly one-third. In other words, two-fifths (40%) of the 30% increase in the number of people wearing eyeglasses is attributable to factors other than population growth.

"While the population 5 to 19 has increased by somewhat better than one-third, the number of eyeglass users in this age group has more than doubled since 1956.

"It is estimated that about two in ten people five years and older who do not wear eyeglasses are in need of glasses today. This comes to approximately 15,000,000 people. The key to getting non-wearers to wear glasses is to motivate them to have their eyes examined.

"Better than one-half of present non-wearers, or approximately 42,000,000 people, probably never had a bona fide eye and vision examination. Nearly one-half of the nonwearers who did have at least one professional eye and vision examination (15,000,000 people) have not had an examination in four years.

"It is estimated that a minimum of 8 in 10 people who do not wear glasses — when submitting to a professional eye examination and given a prescription — will make a purchase.

"It is estimated that approximately 21,000,000 people, that is better than 2 in 10 eyeglass wearers five years and over, are in need of new, updated prescriptions.

"The key to getting eyeglass users to wear up-to-date prescriptions is to motivate them to take more frequent re-examinations.

"Approximately 25,000,000 eyeglass wearers are overdue for re-examination — that is, have not had a professional eye or vision examination in over two and a half years.

"Eight in ten eyeglass wearers who did have their eyes examined during the past two and a half years had their prescription changed.

"It is estimated that of the present 99,000,000 eyeglass wearers five years and older, only approximately 30,000,000 have additional pairs of glasses in their current prescription.

"One of the keys to expansion of additional eyeglass ownership is prescription sunglasses.

"The market for prescription sunglasses is growing. While the number of eyeglass wearers five years and older has increased by nearly one-third since 1956, the number of prescription sunglass owners has better than doubled since that time."

May I suggest that you read these figures over again and study them so that you may properly weigh the implications.

22 Glaucoma

There are many and varied descriptions of what is considered glaucoma. One eye specialist from Pennsylvania puts it this way. "In glaucoma the movement of a fluid that constantly bathes and nourishes the eyes is slowed by the clogging of tiny canals inside the eyeball. Pressure caused by backed-up fluid gradually damages the retina and optic nerve, and results in blindness. It is believed that profound influence of emotion on intra-ocular pressure, does have some effect on the central nervous system."

The following is the generally accepted medical version of glaucoma.

"Glaucoma is an eye condition in which there is an increase of intraocular tension (pressure inside the eye) to a point that causes progressive harm to vision. Although it occurs in many different forms, the primary characteristic of glaucoma is a disturbance in the production and/or drainage of the fluid that fills the inner eye: too great a quantity of fluid may be produced, for example, or a normal amount may not drain properly. These changes may be either slight or intense, periodic or constant in their development. In any case, when too great a pressure is present or when an eye is sufficiently damaged to lose vision, it is said to have glaucoma.

"There are three main types: 1) The acute (narrow angle) kind in which a rapid blocking of the eye drainage system occurs. It comes with little or no warning and is typically accompanied by severe pain, redness of the eye, headache, marked reduction in vision, nausea and vomiting, dilatation of the pupil, and a greenish reflex on shining a light into the eye.

"2) The chronic (open angle) simple type in which a slow, unnoticed, irregular loss of field of view occurs first. In advanced stages central vision is affected.

"3) The secondary kind in which the drainage system of the eye is blocked or impaired by infection, injury, or by a tumor which may be near the drainage canal."

In open angle glaucoma you seldom get a warning nor do you see any symptoms. The vision seems normal and there is seldom any pain or discomfort . . . then suddenly it is too late. The only bit of warning that you get is that your field of vision or peripheral vision gradually diminishes. *So this is your cue. If you find your peripheral vision getting less that is the time to take action.*

The maddening part of open angle glaucoma is the fact that your straight-ahead vision is as good as ever. This is referred to as tunnel or gun barrel vision. Here is what Dr. Banks Anderson of Duke University Medical Center has to say.

"Few diseases require of the patient so much faith in his physician as does open angle glaucoma. The disease is often diagnosed in the absence of symptoms, since early loss of peripheral field and moderate elevation of intraocular pressure usually pass unnoticed. The patient cannot appreciate cupping of his optic disks nor can he measure his intraocular pressure. He must rely on his physician to diagnose and control his disease.

"Miotic drops such as pilocarpine often are required. If central lens opacities are present, this treatment may produce more loss of vision than existed before it was given. Accepting this present loss and discomfort in order to prevent future blindness requires more faith than many persons possess. When one eye is lost, the patient may return as a believer, but advanced atrophy in the remaining eye may make salvage of vision difficult. The complications of surgery for filtering glaucoma are great, but such surgery may be required because of failure to use the medication necessary for control of the disease. Open angle glaucoma is a prevalent disease in the older population. The cornerstones of its control are early diagnosis, careful treatment, and continuing supervision."

I'm giving you Dr. Anderson's full statement so that you'll realize that there isn't too much hope in glaucoma so the thing to do is to prevent it and you can only prevent it by proper nutrition. Of course the eye doctors and the optometrists tell you that the way to help yourself is to have regular eye examinations but I'm telling you . . . change your living habits so that you can prevent glaucoma from ever striking and you'll prevent high blood pressure and heart disease at the same time because it is recognized that there definitely is a link or a relationship between glaucoma and high blood pressure and this information comes to us from two British ophthalmologists, Drs. David A. Leighton and Calbert I. Phillips of the University of Manchester.

Let me also state — what is the use or purpose of going to your eye specialist for regular checkups even if he does find glaucoma or cataract since there is absolutely nothing he can do about it by their own clear-cut admission?

One authority, Dr. Irving Leopold, maintains that "Glaucoma cannot be cured but it can be controlled successfully by medication or surgery if treatment is begun early enough."

Here we have a good description of what happens in the eyes in glaucoma.

"The eye disease glaucoma is usually associated with too much pressure within the eye. Please refer to the diagram in following the description of what occurs in glaucoma.

"Normally the front portion (posterior and anterior chambers) of the eyeball is filled with a circulating fluid (aqueous humor) which is constantly being formed and drained off. In glaucoma this drainage is impaired — the outflow channels do not carry the fluid out of the anterior chamber as they should. (The fluid flow is obstructed in its passage through a pore-like structure to the Canal of Schlemm and on to veins within the sclera.) Pressure begins to build up within the eyeball. This increasing pressure becomes dangerous: Inside the eye, on its back wall, or retina, are thousands of tiny, sensitive nerve cells connected to nerve fibers — and blood vessels, which carry the blood that nourishes them. Increased pressure, by reducing the blood supply, can destroy these retinal nerve cells and their fibers. A certain amount of sight is permanently lost with each cell and fiber destroyed."

Glaucoma usually occurs in persons of middle age or older but it does occasionally turn up in young adults. There appears to be some evidence to indicate that it could possibly have hereditary tendencies. The local accepted causes of glaucoma are obstruction of the angle of the anterior chamber. This apparently brings about the rise of intraocular pressure. But this is definitely not the only or basic cause. It is definitely known that mydriatic drugs are a cause of glaucoma. It is believed that the vitreous solution in the eye for some reason becomes hypertonic in comparison with the blood and absorbs fluid as a result of this. Thus, the absorption of the fluid causes tremendous pressure but the question is, "What causes the vitreous to become hypertonic?"

The commonest manifestation or symptom of glaucoma is blockage of the aqueous outflow channels or a deficiency of the outflow facility. This is termed in medical jargon as Stenosis.

Dr. Paul Courtright Whyte states, "Essentially it means that the eyeball water pressure is too high, with the pressure damaging the sensitive retinal nerves. The water in the eye is the fluid of the body, without the red and white cells, found normally in the blood vessels."

He continues, "The circulation of the body is like the flowing of a river, subject to interference similar to what a dam accomplishes in a river. Regardless, the river keeps on running. Same thing with the fluid circulation of the eye, the outflow of the fluid may be interfered with but this does not reduce the hydraulic interlock which keeps the 'inflow' coming.

"The cell condition of depressed secretion function, labeled glaucoma does not come on overnight. Many years are involved and the condition represents not just trouble in the eye alone but a disturbance over the whole body. The eyes just happen to be the most vulnerable point. Surgery and drug store chemicals may on some occasions save vision as a court of last resort, neither however get to the basic why, which is simply disturbed cell function due to improper 'cause-effect' sequences concerning health."

Many medical men claim that the cause of glaucoma is severe eyestrain or prolonged work under poor lighting conditions. It is also known that a general run-down condition of the patient has something to do with the onset of the trouble. It is believed, however, by naturopathic authorities that the basic cause of glaucoma is very closely aligned with the causes of cataract. There is no question that glaucoma and cataract are toxic conditions brought about by faulty nutrition and wrong general living habits. The medical treatment for glaucoma is usually surgery with the intent of relieving the internal pressure set-up in the eyes as a result of the excess fluid. The only thing that surgery can do is temporarily relieve the pressure.

Dr. Harold M. Peppard describes glaucoma as a condition in which the pressure of the fluids in the eyes increases above the normal to such an extent that it interferes with accommodation. In addition to this interference in accommodation the increased pressure prevents the normal flow of blood to the retina and a gradual degeneration begins. If this is allowed to continue the retina is destroyed and permanent blindness results. The pressure of the fluids in the eyes is kept in balance by their rate of secretion and escape through minute openings. Since any strain on the eye increases the tension of the eye muscles, this fluid balance is interfered with. Because these fluids are not allowed to secrete and escape freely, the pressure in the eye increases.

Glaucoma is a condition in which there is an excess of fluid in the eye which is brought about by faulty eye drainage and congestion of the eye tissues. Many instances of glaucoma have been allowed to continue until there are few if any means to correct the condition. When this happens there are few, if any, forms of treatment that can bring about improvement without surgery. However, drastic changes in dietary and living habits can bring benefits even in advanced stages of glaucoma.

While cataracts are the greatest cause of blindness glaucoma ranks as the second most common cause of loss of vision. It is estimated that more than one and one-half million Americans past the age of 40 have glaucoma. The strange part of this is that at least half of those afflicted don't know they are suffering from glaucoma. The medical profession recommends yearly visits to your eye specialist for tests to detect if eye disorders afflict the patient. The most common symptoms of glaucoma are pain in the eye with the pupils turning gray and cloudy along with faulty peripheral vision. With time the disease progresses until frontal vision also narrows. This usually affects the sufferer so that he sees halos around lights.

Now it is also known that emotion, worry, insomnia and cerebral factors have a predisposing effect in glaucoma. The thalamus which is said to be the seat of emotions has been considered to be the pathological centre of the condition. It is also recognized that starvation and dissipation could be contributory factors. Arteriosclerosis is also known to be an important factor in some cases of glaucoma and it would appear that on occasions the optic atrophy is due to sclerosis of its arterial vessels. Disturbed pituitary function also could be a cause of glaucoma. Also disturbance of the autonomic nervous system may have an effect upon the intraocular pressure. Some imbalance of the autonomic system does occur in many cases of glaucoma. From a medical report it is claimed that as a rule the prognosis is unfavorable. The intraocular tension tends to continue high in spite of all treatment and the majority of patients in whom both eyes are infected become blind.

It is claimed that glaucoma and cataracts are usually accompanied by very low levels of vitamin C in the lens.

267

Extensive medical findings show that vitamin C is closely related to the health of the lens.

Under normal conditions the cornea and the lens are highly and clearly transparent. However, if the blood stream is choked and blocked with wastes and particularly if the blood pressure is high then there is a clear tendency for either of these structures to become misty or cloudy. When the lens is affected it is known as cataract which can usually be seen from the outside as a milky cloudiness behind the pupil. When the pressure of the aqueous humor builds up because of insufficient drainage, a somewhat similar but acutely painful condition results and this is known as glaucoma.

It would appear that the people who drink large quantities of milk seem to have a higher incidence of both cataract and glaucoma. It is claimed that the Jains, a religious sect in India, who drink large quantities of milk have a very high incidence of glaucoma.

A substance known as rutin, which is a component of the old vitamin P, was experimentally administered to a group of patients with glaucoma. Twenty-six patients were treated with 20 milligrams of rutin three times a day. The result — 17 noticed a fall in the pressure inside the eye, 4 claimed that results did not indicate anything definite, while 5 subjects suggested that there was no change at all.

It is believed that approximately 3% of all people over 60 will develop glaucoma. When attacks of glaucoma are only mild they are usually dealt with by physicians using various eye drops. The medical profession considers the underlying cause of glaucoma to be unknown but the symptoms occur because of the inability of the fluid within the eyeball to drain out of the eye at a normal rate. It appears that farsighted people are more prone than nearsighted people to develop glaucoma. One of the earliest symptoms in the development of glaucoma is the appearance of halos around lights. There may also be pain and a sense of fullness in the eyeball.

It has been discovered that glaucoma patients usually exhibit deficiencies of vitamins A, B, C and calcium and various other minerals. Dr. Rolf Ulrich reports a connection between coffee and glaucoma. His patients are all absolutely forbidden the use of coffee. In the paper, Clinical Physiology, (autumn 1962) it is mentioned that glaucoma has been caused by certain antispasmodic drugs. Glaucoma has been known to be caused by doctors themselves when they use steriod drugs injudiciously. Steriods are sometimes put into the eyes by practitioners who are not specialists to treat eye inflammation.

Tobacco may cause constriction of the blood vessels supplying the optic nerve (connecting the retinal cells to the brain), and adversely affect glaucoma.

SURGICAL TREATMENT OF GLAUCOMA

The surgical treatment of glaucoma consists of cutting a hole in the anterior chamber of the eyeball to permit the fluid to drain out under the conjunctiva (the thin membrane covering the white of the eye). The medical profession believes that surgery is effective in preventing blindness when glaucoma has developed. If however, the glaucoma has already resulted in blindness, surgery may not help.

In acute glaucoma, unless the symptoms subside within a few hours, immediate surgery is necessary to save the sight. A piece of iris (the colored portion of the eye) is removed in order to permit fluid to escape from the anterior chamber of the eye. This type of surgery is referred to as an iridectomy.

It is claimed by the medical profession that if surgery is performed before loss of vision has persisted for more than a few hours, about 90 percent of the operations are successful. In chronic glaucoma if the operation is performed before extensive damage has been done to the optic nerve and to vision, most operations are successful. It must be stressed that even after surgery it is necessary to use drug eyedrops to keep the pupils dilated. Remember, this is recommended even after successful surgery.

OTHER TREATMENTS

Various drugs are used in the treatment of glaucoma. One drug, used as drops in the eye, is placed in the eye to keep the pupil constantly contracted. This is believed to permit excess fluid to exit from the eyeball. It is recommended that glaucoma patients or those afflicted with glaucoma should try to avoid emotional upset and should limit their fluid intake. The medical physician usually believes that when it has been established that medical treatment will no longer restrict the pressure in the eyeball to a safe level surgery is advisable.

The drug that is widely used and recommended for the treatment of glaucoma by physicians is known as pilocarpine. It originally came from the leaves of pilocarpus microphyllus but it is now made synthetically. It is very widely used as eye drops but the human toxicity according to Merck states, "Overdoses may produce flushing, diaphoresis, sialorrhea, nausea, vomiting, diarrhoea, tachycardia, miosis. Pulmonary edema may occur in patients with cardiovascular disease."

My advice, calculated and carefully weighed, is that pilocarpine is deadly and dangerous, actually much worse than the condition it is supposed to aid.

A naturopathic physician of my acquaintance claims

excellent results in clearing up or curing glaucoma and cataract by means of fasting and a strict regimen of proper, natural foods which naturopaths claim are blood and lymph purifying. This famous naturopathic physician claims that after a persistent period of at least 6 months on a proper diet glaucoma can be defeated. This physician further states that when they go back to their surgeon or medical practitioner for examination they find that the glaucoma has disappeared. In a specific case of my acquaintance a lady who routinely visited her medical doctor was advised to have surgery for her eyes. However, she tried the naturopathic treatment and it produced results and cleared up her problem completely.

From an article in Optical Developments, published in February 1957, we read, "As enzymes control all our metabolic processes and enzymes are composed of vitamins (or hormones or both), together with minerals and specific proteins, there is opportunity during the constructive stages of life to improve the condition of the eye through enhancing the nutritive values of the diet."

Research has indicated that vitamin C has the ability to reduce the pressure in the eyeball and vitamin C treatment for this condition has been practically 100 percent effective. Heavy doses are required, even as much as 10-15 grams per day, ranging up to even 30 grams per day, in the most severe cases.

In the American Journal of Ophthalmology there was an article by Dr. David O. Harrington. He states that many disturbances and diseases of the eye are partially or completely 'psychogenic' which I presume you know means by the mind. He suggests that greater attention should be paid to emotional problems when a cure is sought. He claims that glaucoma which often leads to total blindness is due to defective circulation in the vessels which supply the blood to the eyes and since circulation is controlled by the central nervous system, emotional conflict may affect it. Hence it is of the greatest importance to first feed the body the materials which are needed to build good healthy eye cells and then to learn to relax and help your mind direct the flow of blood to all affected parts of the body. As long as there is tension and strain the flow of blood to the various organs is impeded.

Dr. Harrington's findings are corroborated by many other top ranking researchers. Therefore, this bit of advice is well worth following.

Generally speaking, medical drug treatment of various types and kinds is tried or given to glaucoma sufferers but if these fail to bring results and often they do fail, then surgery is recommended.

In the American Journal of Ophthalmology of May 1950 Drs. E. V. Omen and F. D. Mossmann gave their experiences with treating patients with serious eye troubles which appeared to be the result of the use of belladonna. From the record it appears that all of the 6 patients had been prescribed belladonna by their physicians. They all had been treated for gastro-intestinal disorders which range from duodenal and peptic ulcers to colitis and hyperacidity. The age range was from 38 to 68 years of age. The ophthalmologists soon learned that all of them had acquired glaucoma. It could not be definitely proven that these 6 patients did not have glaucoma prior to taking belladonna but they did have glaucoma and they all used belladonna.

However, there have been other experiences by physicians with their patients developing glaucoma after using belladonna for any length of time.

When nutritional factors are the cause of glaucoma or cataract — this is frequently the case and in fact, most often the case — to seek improvement or cure by local exercise is just a waste of time. It is generally advised to seek professional advice, be it a medical or a naturopathic physician. Unless you are well informed it is best not to try to doctor your eyes yourself. If you were well informed on health you would not be suffering from this condition. In many cases by following a drastic change in diet and living habits relief from glaucoma can be found. A drastic reduction in starches and liquids in your diet can be of tremendous help, especially such liquids as coffee, tea and alcoholic beverages. If, at the same time, you use only fresh fruits and vegetables the improvement should be more marked. I cannot stress the dietary factors too much. I consider them the most important of all factors pertaining to the eyes in cataract and glaucoma.

Let me quote you a report from a columnist by the name of Durling who was with the Seattle Post-Intelligencer some years ago. "A Berkely, California subscriber says that three eye specialists told him his eyesight was failing so rapidly he would be blind in two years. All the specialists said nothing could be done about it. Then a friend suggested to this man that he try drinking carrot juice. He did. As a result he says his eye condition is completely cured. Not only that, the carrot juice habit seems to have made his hair grow. At any rate he has much more hair than when he started to consume carrot juice regularly".

I would like to quote here the opinion of a qualified optometrist concerning glaucoma.

"About Glaucoma: Anyone who experiences this condition of impaired eye water flow, has earned it fair and square UNLESS it is a genetic condition for which the ancestors and their screwed up nutrition/drugs behavior is responsible. The earning may be innocent but as you know Nature does not excuse stupidity. Those who sleepwalk or get pushed off a ten story building experience the same

273

impact as he who jumps off intentionally. The problem of avoiding glaucoma is the same as the problem of being wise in anything. We are all born totally stupid and too many of us dispell the fog but a little in this direction and that as we age. Wisdom about body care demands reading, study, personal experimentation. Since the schools do such a lousy job of teaching 'whole body' understanding, the individual must make it a do-it-yourself operation. And how many do?''

Here is an interesting article from a book on eyes concerning prevention of glaucoma.

''The prevention of glaucoma is achieved by merely maintaining low intraocular pressure during the lifetime of the individual. The treatment of the disease, once it occurs, is to endeavor to reduce the intraocular pressure to normal levels to prevent further nerve damage. About a million Americans over forty years of age have glaucoma without knowing it. Many cases go undetected for years in spite of the availability of a simple, rapid, and painless tonometer test procedure. Control and prevention of the disease in its early preclinical stages is preferable to waiting for the agony of acute glaucoma to strike.''

The cause and cure of glaucoma seem to be terribly muddled. It is almost inconceivable that in this day and age all the healers cannot seem to handle glaucoma with any satisfactory worthwhile outcome. Obviously glaucoma sufferers have no place to turn, especially if they do not have nutritional knowledge. Frankly, if my eyes were afflicted with glaucoma as of today I would first indulge in a strict fast. Then I would go on to a raw, fresh vegetable and fruit juice diet. I would change my eating habits so that I would be eating mainly raw vegetables, grains and fruits and if the condition had not progressed too far I'd be certain that relief would be forthcoming and the condition would not return as long as I maintained the change.

274

Perhaps this doesn't appear to offer any great hope but on the other hand, it is a great deal more than the medical profession can offer with drugs that do serious, irreparable harm, and surgery that has little or no value except to alleviate your pain and which leaves a scar on the eye forever with diminished functional ability.

It is obvious that the body must be built up, probably from scratch, because where glaucoma has been allowed to develop serious deterioration has set in. Help yourself to relief from glaucoma and also at the same time to better general health by a drastic change in dietary and living habits as suggested.

23 Terminology and Various Errors of Refraction

Emmetropia — When parallel rays are focused exactly on the retina with the eye in a condition of rest, the refraction of the eye is normal or emmetropic and the condition is known as emmetropia.

Ametropia — When, with the eye in a condition of rest, parallel rays are not focused on the retina, but behind or in front of it, the eye is ametropic, and the condition is known as ametropia. The forms of ametropia (errors of refraction) are hypermetropia, myopia, and astigmatism.

Hypermetropia — (or far-sightedness) is that form of ametropia in which the axis of the eyeball is short or the refractive power of the eye weak, so that parallel rays would be brought to a focus behind the retina. Another name for this condition is Hyperopia.

Myopia — (near-sightedness) is that form of ametropia in which the axis of the eyeball is long or the refractive power strong, so that parallel rays are brought to a focus in front of the retina.

Strabismus — A Greek word meaning 'squint' and it describes what is commonly recognized as turned eye(s). This condition is usually caused by imbalance between the eyes. Since the two eyes do not function as a matched team, the ability to see three-dimensionally suffers. A child with uncorrected strabismus, for example, will be handicapped in precision work requiring binocular coordination. Incidentally, when I was a boy we called this condition "cock-eye".

Presbyopia — Caused by a gradual loss of focusing ability that is normal for everyone. When the focusing ability of an individual's eyes has decreased to the point where vision at his reading distance becomes blurry and difficult, the condition is known as presbyopia. This generally occurs between the ages of 40 and 45. A need to hold reading material further away or symptoms of 'eyestrain' (headache, fatigue, or concentration difficulty) while doing close work may be caused by presbyopia. This condition is generally referred to as old age sight. It's when your arms become too short to hold the reading matter. That is, you have to move it away so that you can see it. This indicates loss of elasticity or accommodation.

Astigmatism — is that form of ametropia in which the refraction in the several meridians of the eyeball is different. The "a" means without, while "stigma" means point. Thus, it is an optical system without a point of focus, or as Webster puts it "A structural defect of a lens, or an eye, that prevents light rays from an object from meeting in a single focal point, so that indistinct images are formed."

Eye coordination — In order to have good vision, you must not only see clearly with each eye, but both eyes must also be able to simultaneously point or aim at the same object — quickly, easily, and automatically. Your eyes must work together as a team. If they do not, you (1) will

278

see double, or (2) must disregard or block out the image seen by one eye, or (3) must make an additional effort to force both eyes to point at the same object at the same time.

Amblyopia — is a term used for unexplained reduction of visual acuity (clearness of vision). "Unexplained" means that, even with proper corrective lenses and in the absence of detectable eye disease, the acuity of the eye is still below normal. Amblyopia almost always affects only one eye. It is generally agreed that this eye must have best correctable visual acuity of 20/40 or less to be considered amblyopic. Only central vision is affected by amblyopia. Peripheral vision (side vision) is unaffected.

In normal vision the six extrinsic muscles all operate in unison and at equal tension and with equal strength so that the eyeball remains symmetrical in shape.

For more than 100 years far-sightedness, short-sightedness and astigmatism have been conditions which the medical profession and the eye specialists tell us absolutely nothing can be done about except to prescribe glasses . . . and this applies to children, too. It's a rather dim prospect for a child or a young person afflicted with any one of these three conditions.

When it happens in a child it is accepted that the condition is congenital which means it was contributed to by the parents. However, frequently the child is born with normal vision and normal eyes but any one of these conditions develop. Then there is nothing that the medical profession can do to correct the condition except to prescribe glasses.

The following comes from the Merck Index.

"Corrective therapy consists of the prescribing of

279

suitable lenses to compensate for the refractive errors found by a skilled ophthalmologist."

It appears that for various reasons we allow our eyes to become lazy. Also, I am suspicious or fearful that the intake of cow's milk in our infancy, childhood and youth is a contributing factor in the development of these three conditions. It is my sincere belief that glasses should never be prescribed at least until some attempt has been made to correct the condition by nutrition and by means of exercise.

Optometrists and ophthalmologists believe that errors of refraction can only be corrected by prescribing or providing glasses. It is obviously not the desire or intent of the profession to provide ways or means of correcting errors of refraction by any other means than eye crutches. It is just too lucrative to do it any other way.

24 Summary

From the moment... some three years ago... I started seeking and gathering information on cataract for this book I was determined that I would leave no stone unturned to learn everything humanly possible about cataracts... cause, contributing factors and cure if humanly possible. At this moment I'm trying to sum up what I have learned and judging by everything that I have read on the subject — and I have searched everywhere — I think I know as much about it as any other investigator and probably a lot more.

It has long been established by those interested in health, be they scientists or laymen, that you can't have a healthy mind in a sick body anymore than you can have a sick mind in a healthy body. The same rule holds true for the eyes. You can't have sick eyes in a healthy body and you can't have a healthy body if you have sick eyes. I maintain that nutrition is still the key to eye health just as it is to health of the mind and of the body.

After intensive, extensive studies I cannot help but

feel that senile cataract is due to nutritional imbalance and deficiency, the supply and drainage routes being impaired, resulting in the clouding of the lens.

If, as of the time you are reading this book you do not have cataract or glaucoma, then by following the common sense, practical advice given herein you need never fear cataract or glaucoma. I mean this with all my heart and I ask you to believe me. The advice given in this book is sound, practical and scientific. From my studies diet is not the only factor in cataracts but it is by far the most important factor.

If you already have cataracts but they have not reached the end-of-the-trail stage where surgery is practically imminent or unavoidable then you can still attack the cataracts by changing your way of life. Furthermore, the development can be stopped in its tracks and by continuing the advice and directions contained herein, you can improve the condition until the cataracts disappear. I have quoted letters and references in this book that clearly prove what I say is true and that it is possible to stop cataracts and make them disappear.

When cataracts have developed to what is known as the ripe stage or complete opacity you are, by generally accepted standards, blind. Therefore, there is little else left except surgical removal of the lens to be followed by the lens built into the glasses that will be provided for you. With the aid of these glasses you can see quite well once you have adjusted to them and life will be liveable. Of course, you will only be able to see straight ahead but it is still a lot better than being blind with the ripe cataracts. With contact lenses it is claimed that you also have peripheral vision but then I must warn you contacts often create more problems than they correct.

I feel that the term "ripening" as used by the medical

profession in the past and also in the present should be explained. It does not mean what many might expect it to mean . . . something like maturity or a natural progression. What is actually meant is that you continue to go to your doctor and keep on doing the things you have been doing like violating natural biological principles and abusing your eyes and not nourishing them properly. This will in time create complete opacity in your lens which means "blindness". Then you go back to your surgeon and he will perform the surgery and remove the opaque lens. This is what is meant by "ripening" and the operation is called Surgical Extraction of the eye lens.

To me it is unjust for the medical profession to advise people with cataracts to sit and let them develop until they are ripe and then advise surgery for removal. I think it is just as unfair to perform surgery on an eye that has not developed cataract to any great degree because the other eye does have a cataract. However, that is the way they advocate doing it now so that you won't have to go through the trauma of having one eye done and then waiting until the other eye is "ripe" and in the meantime having your vision terribly upset. I repeat, it is tragic that the great and noble medical profession has to resort to this type of chicanery when there definitely are other methods that have proved and are proving successful in improving the vision and correcting the condition as I have clearly outlined in this book.

From the accumulated evidence it is absolutely clear that cataract is fundamentally or basically a deficiency disease and also the specifically deficient vitamins are mainly riboflavin (B2) and also A, C, D and E. As I have illustrated also in this book, there are differences of opinion from various researchers concerning the research and experimental work that brought about the conclusion that riboflavin deficiency was definitely a cause of cataract. Probably I am the first man to point out that when the

283

riboflavin was not conclusively proven to correct the condition it was due to the fact that the riboflavin was not provided along with other essential vitamins or nutrients. For example, in conjunction with adequate quantities of vitamin A.

I have been studying nutrition for 20 years and I was one of the first researchers to point out that to prescribe or give specific, single vitamins to correct a condition was absolutely in error. Vitamins do not act or fulfill their function alone. They work only or best along with other vitamins and substances. Therefore, I again make it clear and straight that it is my firm conviction — and there is more than substantial proof available — that cataract is caused by a deficiency of mainly riboflavin and A, C, D and E and can, in practically every case, be corrected by a supply of these vitamins provided the condition has not been permitted to progress to a terminal state. Furthermore, the riboflavin must be supplied in a form that is readily assimilable and metabolizable by the body, preferably in conjunction with vitamin A.

As you may glean from my writing I research researchers and their research. I study the work that they have done and analyze their work. Then I make my findings based upon their work. Furthermore, whereas one researcher is concerned only with his single project I am studying and investigating literally hundreds of research projects along the same lines as this one researcher.

Now I'd like to point out that normally riboflavin is not absent in the diet but somehow when the amount of riboflavin stored or held in the body goes below a certain figure the body does not release any more riboflavin. Research projects have proven this to be true. In other words, while the eyes and other parts of the body suffered due to a lack of riboflavin yet upon autopsy it was found that the body did contain minimal quantities of this vitamin and research has thus established that there is a minimal basic quantity that the body will not release.

Furthermore, I have a feeling that there are many substances which are taken into the body as food or medicine that cause the riboflavin to be wasted or to be rendered unassimilable. This was clearly demonstrated in a research project that pinpointed galactose, a substance derived from milk, as an antagonist of riboflavin. It is also a fact, however, that dairy products in themselves contain and contribute riboflavin to the body but here again a mysterious atmosphere prevails. While the dairy products contain riboflavin and it is thus available to the body, when the dairy products are ingested the body still suffers from a deficiency of this vitamin. This illustrates that in the processing or in treatment or commercialization of the dairy product something occurs which renders the riboflavin either unassimilable or causes it to be wasted.

My studies reveal that in visual problems with children, pasteurized milk is involved. Before allowing glasses to be prescribed for a child first I beg you eliminate all forms of milk from the child's diet. Don't let that frighten you. There are plenty, plenty of good foods without milk. Many children cannot take milk. So try and eliminate milk when the doctor prescribes glasses for your child. Try it for a few weeks and you may find that by eliminating milk or all dairy products that the child's vision will become normal again and thus he won't need the glasses.

As galactose is a form of sugar I am suggesting that the use of sugar in the normal diet is a factor, perhaps a comprehensive factor in cataract. Remember, the sugar that we use in our diet is refined sugar and because it has most of its elements and minerals removed I suggest that it actually leaches various elements from the body or causes them to be locked up and rendered unavailable.

285

While I cannot prove that sugar is a factor I feel certain that it is a contributing factor in cataract and I'm suggesting to any cataract sufferer, immediately eliminate all forms of sugar. Now I did not say all forms of sweetening, I said sugar. You still have honey and fruits to act as sweeteners. Furthermore, from various pieces of evidence that I have gathered, I have learned something else and I want to make this statement clear. Any person who smokes or drinks alcoholic beverages cannot have good eyesight. I mean this seriously and not because I'm trying to attack these vices. I feel positive that both smoking and drinking do seriously affect the eyes.

I'm clearly attacking the medical profession, the ophthalmologists, the opticians and the optometrists for their part in advising the use of glasses. The optical companies have for at least 40 years bribed the medical profession, the ophthalmologists and others by giving them kickbacks in the form of huge cheques for the number of glasses that they prescribe. Remember, this kickback is in addition to the high fees charged by the eye specialists and those engaged in various phases of the profession or business. Back in the 40's it was known that more than 3,000 eye doctors in the U.S.A. were receiving kickbacks or bribes from the optical companies. There is no reason to believe that the situation has been entirely corrected. That is why glasses are prescribed almost 100 percent to people who visit these practitioners or consult them. I suggest glasses are prescribed whether they are needed or not and in places where the eyes are close to normal very weak or window clear glasses are prescribed and that is why no permanent corrective measures are ever suggested or recommended.

I strongly advise against the use of contact lens. I contend the only justification for contact lens is cosmetic purposes. Maybe if you're an actor or in some profession where it wouldn't be nice to wear glasses, then perhaps there is some justification for the use of contact lens. Otherwise, I say never use them. I still believe that 95% of all the glasses prescribed can be avoided if the nutritional problems are corrected. It is obvious that the medical and optometrical professions do not seek the cause of the conditions they treat. They are only interested in correction by drugs and surgery and I add also because these sources pay off well.

I firmly assert that by following the clear advice and directions given in this book both cataract and glaucoma can be prevented . . . there is not the faintest doubt in my mind, I stress and repeat that both of these conditions are unnecessary and, by following my counsel, can be prevented.

Here I will go a step further and state that if the situation is recognized and caught in the early stages before it reaches an advanced state you can definitely make it recede and cause the cloudiness to disappear in cataract. I fully realize that this is in distinct contradiction to the statements and opinions of the medical profession that both cataract and glaucoma cannot be cured without drastic surgery. Of course, I want to emphasize that what the medical profession calls cure by surgery is not a cure at all or in any sense of the word. You cannot cure an organ or a condition by removing the organ. It is like telling you that you can remove a limp in your leg by removing the leg. I suggest that removing the lens is in a similar category.

The reason the medical profession claim that both cataract and glaucoma cannot be cured is because they have never experimented with or tried natural therapy. I've always given the same reason for their refusal to try natural therapy . . . because it would drastically reduce their earning power and their revenue. After all is said and done, if they preach the doctrine of natural therapy the average individual would immediately say "Who needs a doctor when nature performs her own miracle at no cost?" ... because nature does not charge a fee, she only requests or demands obedience which, if followed, brings the desired results.

Where no accident or occupational hazards are involved normal healthy people do not develop cataract, glaucoma or other eye disorders.

As I study the whole bizzare picture of cataract, glaucoma and various eye conditions plus the recommendations and opinions of optometrists, ophthalmologists and opticians I find that each in turn stresses the importance of regular visits to his specific kind of guidance or treatment. It appears they are all in the same position as the medical profession where they urge the individual to visit the physician or the practitioner of their choice frequently.

It is my humble opinion that good nutrition and proper health habits are far, far more important than visits to your MD, OD or any other healer, be it for your eyes or other parts of your anatomy.

It is my positive conclusion that without nutritional guidance and acceptance little if any progress can be made in the care of the eyes or the correction or prevention of glaucoma and cataract. The medical profession admit boldly that drugs cannot help these conditions or are totally ineffective. Exercise no doubt is beneficial but without proper nutrition there is no possibility of benefitting the eyes or treating or curing cataract, glaucoma or other disorders. Therefore, I stress that if you want help for your eyes you must use nutritional means and methods and this is made crystal clear in this book.

The medical profession perpetuates the myth that as we grow older our organs grow weaker, harden, undergo changes, atrophy and just waste away. And of course that is what they say about our eyes and claim that old age is the main cause of cataract. They put it this way "the eye tissue which is most symptomatic of your passing years is the crystalline lens". In youth the lens is soft and pliable and readily changes and adjusts to accommodate visual needs but in your later years this process becomes less and less functional, eventually leading to various eye conditions, detached retina, glaucoma, cataract and other manifestations of impaired vision. So they prescribe glasses and as the months and years go by these have to be altered or strengthened and this is usually every two years or less and as you get older this changes so that you have to see your eye doctor every year and sometimes even more often.

For glaucoma my advice is prevention because when the onslaught occurs it is usually too late. With cataract at least you can do something when you learn that cataracts are forming but with glaucoma it appears to be a different story. So therefore the answer to glaucoma appears to be mainly prevention.

I realize that the medical profession makes surgery for cataracts sound so very easy but I'm warning you it is not easy, it only sounds easy. If it were easy there wouldn't be so many suicides after cataract surgery or so many bitterly disappointed and disconsolate people.

If you are willing to work at it and to strive to regain your eyesight then you will take the advice that I have given and follow a comparatively Spartan diet and way of life. Lest you feel sorry for yourself, I might add that after a short period you will find that there are so many great benefits that you will be ashamed of yourself for not recognizing the many bounties that this way of life has to offer, apart from the improvement in or the restoration of your vision and the absence of pain and suffering. But this

289

method is not for the weak, not for the servile or the puny. If you have what it takes I sincerely believe that you can regain your vision and your general health. It is strictly up to you whether or not you retain your eyesight or join the half million or so blind or near blind people in America.

Remember, remember, remember, cataracts and glaucoma can be readily prevented. They can be stopped and they can be cured.

BIBLIOGRAPHY

VOLUMES

Adler's Physiology Of The Eye; *Robert A. Moses.*

Better Eyes Without Glasses; *Gayelord Hauser.*

Better Eyesight Without Glasses; *W.H. Bates, M.D.*

Better Sight Without Glasses; *Harry Benjamin.*

Biochemistry Of Disease; *O. Bodansky, M. Bodansky.*

Bionomy Of Power, The; *John X. Loughran.*

Cataract; *Benedict Lust.*

Complete Book Of Vitamins; *Rodale.*

Feel Like A Million; *Catharyn Elwood.*

Food And Life; *Yearbook Of Agriculture 1939, U.S. Government.*

Get Well Naturally; *Linda Clark.*

Handbook Of Food And Agriculture; *Reinhold Publ. Corporation.*

Healing Power Of Herbs, The; *May Bethel.*

Honey And Your Health; *Bodog F. Beck and Doree Smedley.*

Human Anatomy; *Jackson.*

Improve Your Eyes At Home; *R. Brooks Simpkins.*

Improve Your Sight Naturally; *C. Leslie Thomson.*

Improve Your Sight Without Glasses; *Science of Life Book Pty. Ltd. 1946.*

Let's Get Well; *Adelle Davis.*

Marvels And Oddities Of Sunlight, The; *William J. Fielding.*

May And Worth's Manual of Diseases of the Eye; *T. Keith Lyle and A. G. Cross.*

Merck Index Of Chemicals And Drugs, The; *Merck & Co., Inc.*

Merck Manual; *Eleventh Edition.*

Natural Way To Better Eyesight, The; *J. I. Rodale.*

Near Sight, Aged Sight; *William White Cooper.*

New Breed Of Doctor, A; *Alan H. Nittler, M.D.*

Nutrition; *Chaney and Ahlborn.*

Nutrition And Diet In Health And Disease; *McLester.*

Oculopathy; *R. Brooks Simpkins.*

Overfed But Undernourished; *Dr. Curtis Wood.*

Principles Of Internal Medicine; *Second Edition.*

Quick Guide To Better Vision; *Margaret Darst Corbett.*

Science Of Nutrition Simplified, The; *Rosenwarne.*

See Without Glasses; *Ralph J. MacFadyen.*

Sight Without Glasses; *Dr. Harold M. Peppard.*

Strengthening The Eyes; *Bernarr Macfadden.*

Strong Healthy Eyes Without Glasses; *Dr. R. A. Richardson.*

Taber's Cyclopedic Medical Dictionary.

Textbook Of Biochemistry; *E. Staunton West and W. R. Todd.*

Textbook Of Physiology; *Dr. M. Foster.*

Vitamins: A Survey Of Present Knowledge; *Medical Research Council G.B.*

Vitamins, A Symposium, The; *The American Medical Association.*

Vitamins And Other Dietary Essentials; *Aykroyd.*

Vitamins In Medicine, The; *Bicknell and Prescott.*

Water Of Life; *Armstrong.*

What Must I Do?; *Vanguard Research Ltd.*

Yearbook Of Agriculture; *1959.*

You And Your Eyes; *Lawrence Lewison.*